The presentations of clinical psychiatry

The presentations of clinical psychiatry

by
Robert M Cohen

Quay Books Division, Mark Allen Publishing Group
Jesses Farm, Snow Hill, Dinton, Wiltshire, SP3 5HN

British Library Cataloguing-in-Publication Data
A catalogue record is available for this book

© Robert Cohen 2000
ISBN 1 85642 103 1

Printed in the UK by Redwood Books, Trowbridge, Wilts, UK

Contents

Acknowledgements

This book is written after years of training and studying in psychiatry and is intended as an introduction to the subject. The thoughts in this book arise from many hours spent with patients, psychiatrists who have taught me and those trainee doctors, nurses and others who have given me the opportunity to teach them. There are numerous papers to be obtained if one is to build up a knowledge of a subject: many medical librarians, especially Mrs Stephanie Armstrong at the now closed Friern Hospital, Mrs E Pumphrey at Highlands Hospital, Mr Paul Valentine at West London Healthcare NHS Trust, and Miss Elizabeth Nokes, assisted by Margaret Daly and Dr Cheryl Twomey, at the Library of the Royal College of Psychiatrists, have been particularly kind and helpful. To all these people I extend my grateful thanks.

Much personal time has been expended in writing this book and for their forbearance and constant support throughout the project, I once again thank my wife Liz and my children Tony and Hannah.

Acknowledgements

Caution to the reader

While every effort has been taken in the preparation of this manuscript to ensure reasonable coverage of the subject matter and accuracy of references, the author accepts no responsibility for loss arising out of such errors that might subsequently be found in the book.

The material in this book may form the basis for clinical practice, but all information should be interpreted in the light of the reader's clinical experience. Where the reader is uncertain, he or she should seek advice from a suitably qualified practitioner.

In particular, the reader is advised that the author makes no claim to legal qualification. Where the text refers to legal matters, advice from a qualified lawyer should be sought before action is taken.

Introduction

This is a new type of book introducing psychiatry. Unlike a textbook that describes diseases, in this book, the reader is invited to imagine the interview with a patient. Countless non-psychiatric doctors have suggested to their patients that they might like to 'have a chat' with a psychiatrist, as though it were some frivolous enterprise to be undertaken so that something can be seen to be done, even if they expect it to achieve nothing.

But an interview with a psychiatrist is not the same as a chat with a friend over a cup of coffee. Of course, the interview should be carried out courteously and the patient should feel respected and valued as a person. But the skill of the psychiatrist is to carry out a **formal** and **structured** interview to elicit very specific information. On the basis of this, the psychiatrist will come to the opinion that the patient is (or is not) likely to be suffering from a psychiatric disorder, ie. will make a diagnosis.

In this respect, the psychiatrist is solving problems no differently from other people. Imagine that someone were to come and tell you that he is a solicitor. You might ask him why he claimed to be a solicitor, and he might say that he has worked for a law firm for the last 20 years. That is information he gives you. It is his word and you either believe it or you do not. You might then notice that he wearing a suit and you may consider a suit to be appropriate clothing for a solicitor. Alternatively, if he was wearing dirty blue overalls and had earrings in both ears, and if his hands were covered in oil, you might find his dress strange for a solicitor. It could be that he is a car mechanic, pretending to be a solicitor; it could be that he is a solicitor who enjoys tinkering around with cars in his spare time. If it really mattered and you were looking for a solicitor for a legal case, you might ring up the Law Society to find if he is registered with the Law Society as a solicitor — in English law, this is the definition of what a solicitor is.

On the basis of this (and other similar information, such as his behaviour, the way he talks, the place that you see him) you would come to an opinion about whether this man was, or was not, a solicitor. You would have done three things:

1.   Taken information from the man (his claim to be a solicitor);

2.   Made your own observations (about his dress, how he conducted himself);

3.   Carried out checks to confirm or refute your belief (telephoned the Law Society).

However brief or thorough your enquiries, you would form a judgement. There would be no right and wrong (unless there is a definition; in this case, there is). If the matter is important, you might take exhaustive steps to be certain; if unimportant, you might content yourself with the person's word. And however detailed your enquiries are, there will be times when, in the light of subsequent information, you get it wrong.

Doctors carry out essentially the same procedure to find out information which will help form an opinion about whether a person does or does not have a medical condition. Psychiatry is a branch of medicine, and so the procedures are essentially the same. Doctors:

1. Take information from the patient (what the patient is complaining of) — the **history**;

2. Make their own observations (physical or mental state examination) — the **examination**;

3. As far as possible, carry out checks to confirm or refute their belief (gather information from others; perform blood tests, take X-rays, etc) — the **investigations**.

On the basis of this, the doctor will either conclude that he cannot find any evidence for a medical disorder (this does not mean that the patient does not have an illness, but that if any illness is present, it is not showing itself clearly enough to be detected); or will come to the opinion that a disorder is likely to be present. At this stage, the doctor makes a **diagnosis**, which is a medical opinion of what is likely to be the cause of the patient's discomfort, but is always open to revision in the light of further information.

What makes the medical interview a specialist task is that there are tried and tested ways of conducting it. The history, examination and investigations focus on pieces of information that are known to be relevant to various disease processes. In this book, the process is shown for 10 clinical pictures that are amongst the most common to be seen by psychiatrists (alcoholism; anorexia nervosa; anxiety disorders; dementia; depression; hypomania; mental handicap; obsessive-compulsive disorder; personality disorder [antisocial] and schizophrenia). For each of these pictures, a chapter is presented in three sections:

1. A list of the numerous points that psychiatrists should seek when interviewing a patient, in their appropriate place in the interview, and also points about managing the condition;

2. An essay introducing the psychiatric disorder, to make the disorder more easily understandable to a person who may never or only infrequently have come across people with the condition;

3. A second essay in which some of the medical and scientific research literature that underpins the practice of clinical psychiatry is presented.

The psychiatric interview

When carried out thoroughly, the psychiatric interview is an exhaustive review of the patient's symptoms, background (life history, including enquiry into the family of origin, and current social circumstances), and current mental functioning. The interview can take between two and three hours to complete (although very experienced practitioners can sometimes reduce this to one hour), and given resource limitations in most health services, short cuts may have to be taken. In this case, it is important for the practitioner to know what should be included, even if he or she knows that certain pieces of information that are of less importance may at times be omitted.

In English practice, the format that has become widely accepted is colloquially referred to as a *Maudsley History*. Full details can be found in the book *The Maudsley Handbook of Practical Psychiatry* (edited by Goldberg D, Oxford Medical Publications, 1998), but the main headings are as follows:

- History of presenting complaint
- Family history
- Personal history
- Past medical history
- Past psychiatric history
- Drug history
- pre-morbid personality
- Social circumstances
- Psychosexual history
- Mental state examination
- Investigations
- Management.

History of presenting complaint

In this section, the patient's account of the symptoms are recorded. Although the patient may give the symptoms in a random order, it is the job of the clinician to organise them chronologically and to select, from what the patient says, those comments that are medically relevant for inclusion and exclude those facts that, while being recognised as important to the patient, have no medical relevance.

The clinician should begin at the time when the patient first noticed that something was wrong, describe how things progressed from there and what precipitated the request for medical help. In the case of a chronic condition (as many psychiatric conditions are), it is helpful to summarise the progress from the onset of the disease to the period of relative stability just prior to the present episode of illness.

Family history

The patient is asked to describe the family in which he grew up. Details of each family member, their personality, occupation, medical and psychiatric illnesses (including cause of death) are sought. The aim is to estimate the genetic contribution to the patient's mental disorder and to gain some understanding of the environment in which the patient grew up.

Personal history

In this section the interviewer attempts to chart the patient's life history in chronological order. Details are asked about the patient's birth and early development, school career and work history. Some psychiatrists will ask about personal relationships at this point, others leave it until the psychosexual history. The aim is to see a pattern of behaviour that is repeated (eg. frequent dismissals from work, which may give an insight into an aspect of the patient's character), or to notice an abrupt change (eg. a high-flying career, followed by a period of inexplicable unemployment, suggesting the possibility that an illness has developed).

Past medical history

Details of all previous and current physical illnesses are sought, as these may be affecting the mental state of the patient or even be the cause of the mental illness (eg. hypothyroidism as a cause of depressive illness).

Other illnesses may be found that may be due to a deterioration in lifestyle as a result of mental illness (eg. scurvy in someone who is homeless) or may be a complication of the mental illness (eg. jaundice as a result of alcohol-induced liver damage).

Past psychiatric history

Details are sought mainly of previous episodes of the main mental illness (eg. previous episodes of acute psychosis in schizophrenia), finding out whether the patient has been admitted to hospital (either voluntarily or compulsorily under the provisions of the Mental Health Act 1983), what treatment the patient has had and whether it helped to improve his/her condition or not.

Sometimes two mental disorders occur together.

Drug history

All the medication that the patient is taking should be carefully documented. If the patient has bottles of medication with labels, these should be brought to the interview, so that the name of the medication and the prescribed dose can be accurately recorded. Even medication prescribed for non-psychiatric conditions should be recorded as many of these can cause pictures of mental illness.

The interviewer is advised to enquire carefully about any history of allergic reactions.

Pre-morbid personality

The personality is the pattern of behaviour that the patient has shown repeatedly. For example, the patient may show a propensity to lose his/her temper easily. These patterns are thought to be present since adolescence. In some mental disorders, the patient can appear to change personality as a result of the illness: it is important to be aware of the personality before illness to compare. This information is often best obtained from informants who know the patient well (eg. a spouse, close friend).

Specific enquiry is made about interests and hobbies, religious beliefs and practices, forensic history (where this is thought to be particularly important, this may be a separate section) and use of psychoactive substances, including legal substances such as tobacco and alcohol as well as use of illicit drugs.

Social circumstances

Enquiry is made about the patient's current social situation in respect of employment, accommodation, marital and financial status. In helping the unemployed patient, enquiry should be made about benefits received, as much distress can be alleviated by ensuring that patients in financial difficulties (especially if they are a result of the illness) are receiving all the benefits to which they are entitled. Although the doctor will refer the patient to a social worker to assist with the practicalities of obtaining unclaimed benefits, a doctor who has concern for the welfare of his/her patient will want to include this check.

Psychosexual history

Details are sought of all personal relationships that the patient has had. The patient should be asked about sexual orientation and answers treated with respect. Do not moralise. The patient should be asked for details of all serious partners, the age difference, the partner's occupation, the nature and the length and permanence of the relationships.

The aim of this section is to find out the patterns of relationships selected by the patient (eg. brief relationships with violent partners), the quality of any current support and the nature of stressors such as responsibility for very young children.

Mental state examination

Prior to the mental state examination, the interviewer has asked the patient (and others) for information. The mental state examination is that part of the interview in which the doctor makes his own observations.

Each person provides information about himself in the way that he looks and behaves. The interviewer should, therefore, carefully examine the appearance and behaviour of the patient for clues that suggest the possibility of a psychiatric disorder. The interviewer enquires about the patient's experience of his mood ('mood') and compares this with his own observations of the patient's mood ('affect'). These may agree, but not always, such as in incongruity of affect that is noted at times in some patients with schizophrenia. The interviewer pays attention to the speed, volume, grammar and content of the patient's speech, seeking for abnormalities that suggest abnormal mental processes.

The interviewer makes specific enquiry about suicidal thoughts and plans that the patient may entertain. Questions are asked about the patient's self-esteem, presence or absence of ideas of guilt, and attitude to the future (optimistic or pessimistic). The patient is asked about any unusual ideas or beliefs that may or may not have been already expressed in the interview, and the interviewer tests whether any such beliefs meet the criteria for description as a delusion (a false fixed belief, not in keeping with the patient's cultural background). The patient is asked about the presence or absence of hallucinations and other abnormal mental experiences such as first rank symptoms of schizophrenia. If any abnormal beliefs or experiences are uncovered, an assessment is made by the examiner to determine whether or not the patient has any recognition of the abnormality of his mental experiences (assessment of insight).

The patient is tested as to his cognitive state, to see if there is any evidence of, for example, disorientation or memory impairment.

Investigations

After the history and mental state examination have been completed, the interviewer has reached the limit of the knowledge he can gain from the examination of the patient. A hypothesis of the presence or absence of mental disorder, and possible diagnoses, should now be possible. The interviewer may wish to test this hypothesis by further investigations. A most important step is to gain further information from other people who have observed the patient, such as relatives and friends. It is also very useful to review the medical case notes of the patient. Occasionally, medical investigations such as blood tests, X-rays, CT and MRI scans and EEGs are useful.

Management

This is the part of the interview in which the interviewer offers the patient advice. There may be a suggestion that information is insufficient and the patient may be asked to carry out some task, such as keeping a food diary if anorexia nervosa is suspected or diagnosed, or just reviewed again before a decision can be made about how best to proceed. The advice may be for treatment that will significantly affect the symptoms of the mental disorder or it may be something to ease the situation even if it does not effect a cure. The two types of advice can be given simultaneously. Treatment may involve the administration of some physical entity, such as a medication or ECT; psychological therapy, such as cognitive-behaviour therapy; social therapy, such as rehousing or attendance at a day centre; or it may be a combination of all three of these types of approach, depending on the severity of the disorder and the resources available to provide the treatment.

In this book, there are ten common presentations. The information relevant to the clinical interview is presented in its appropriate place in each chapter. This section is in note form, as an aide-mémoire. Readers should be aware that there are certain conditions where specific information is either not relevant to a section or is not available. In this case, the section may be omitted in that part of that chapter.

The introductory essay

Human behaviour is taken so much for granted that we sometimes lose sight of what is happening. As a result, behaviour that is abnormal can be regarded with fear. Mental disorders are, therefore, often hard to understand for people with little or no previous experience of such disorders in their friends or relatives. In this section of each chapter, an attempt is made to describe the condition in plain, non-technical language. Where it is important to gain this knowledge, certain technical terms or groupings of symptoms are explained more fully.

The **Further reading** referred to in this section is aimed at the general doctor or other health professional, although others without professional training may find these references of interest.

The background literature essay

The current fashion is for 'evidence-based medicine', where the apparently 'new' concept that medicine should be based on evidence is recommended.

Medicine in the western (Hippocratic) tradition has always been a scientific discipline. Doctors are encouraged to observe the illnesses of their patients and evaluate, honestly, the responses of their patients to the treatments tried. Psychiatry is no different and a large literature base has grown up. This ranges from clinical descriptions, through case reports to evaluations of large series. The factors that contribute to the causes of mental illness are sought through epidemiological and basic scientific studies, and treatments are evaluated by observations of response; the most suitable being in the form of a double-blind, randomised, controlled trial. Not every possible question for every possible clinical situation has been answered, and there are times when a course of action needs to be tried despite the absence of scientific underpinning. But this should not discount the comprehensive literature source that has developed around the world.

It would, of course, be ideal if every practitioner could read every piece of research written about his given field. This is impossible as the literature is too vast and often inaccessible even for a person studying it full-time. The task is even more unrealistic for a busy clinician. However, this book does try to assist the clinician. It focuses on the issues that arise in the course of clinical interviewing and management. No attempt is made to review the basic sciences as they apply to psychiatry; there are other books available that provide this information. Here, the reader will find an essay pointing him towards a number of papers in the literature that make a contribution to providing a more firm basis for a piece of clinical practice. But this is not a review essay, and no attempt is made to provide the answer to every possible query. It is hoped that if the clinician pursues some of the references in these chapters, he or she will acquire a good basis to his/her practice, and as the practitioner becomes more experienced in psychiatry, he or she will add to this from his/her own reading.

The intention is that the reader should be able to follow up these references. The majority of doctors do not practise in teaching hospitals with well-endowed libraries. Rather, they are able to access a few general medical and specialist journals. The doctor will be aware that there are relevant and important articles in these journals, but will not find it easy access them. Time available to carry out a search may be limited so, even if located, the articles may remain unread.

This book tries to mirror that reality. On the whole, articles that pertain to psychiatry have been sought in four general medical journals (*British Medical Journal*, *Lancet*, *Journal of the American Medical Association*, *New England Journal of Medicine*) and four general psychiatric journals (*British Journal of Psychiatry*, *Psychological Medicine*, *American Journal of Psychiatry*, *Archives of General Psychiatry*). It is hoped that the majority of doctors in the UK, and a number of others in other countries (especially English-speaking countries), will have access either to the original articles or at least relatively easy and inexpensive access through a local medical librarian. Occasionally, reference is made to a source elsewhere, if the article is of particular importance. It is recognised that the limitation will necessarily distort the choice of articles and subjects covered in accordance with the biases of the individual journals, but the tendency for these journals to provide review articles relatively often gives the reader the opportunity to gain a reasonable degree of coverage.

One particular note of caution for readers, in respect of the literature: the aim of this book is to make the literature more accessible. It is not to evaluate that literature. Readers following up references may find that articles provide less information than expected (eg. a report of two cases, rather than an extensive review of the literature on a topic). Rather than being disappointed, the reader should recognise that this may be the full extent of available information. It is the evidence that will be used in practice, but at least readers will be aware of the limitation of its applicability before a clinical decision is made.

How to use this book

It is hoped the book will be of use to a wide variety of people. Many will be doctors, but it can be of use to other professionals and lay persons. Different people may use the book in different ways.

Senior psychiatrists (consultants and specialist registrars)

Senior psychiatrists should, in theory, know the entire contents of this book and much more besides. However, they may find it useful in two ways:

1.   In a medico-legal setting, this book may help to provide the first few references to back up specialist advice given in court, while further research is being undertaken;

2.   As a teaching aid for use with doctors in training. I have found the first parts of these essays useful as a way of encouraging doctors new to psychiatry to learn much information in a brief space of time and as a revision aid for doctors approaching the MRCPsych examination.

Junior psychiatrists and general practitioners

Those with less experience in psychiatry may find the book useful as a quick introduction. **The psychiatric examination** section provides considerable information in a brief space, as a way of giving an overview and also as a platform on which to base later, more detailed reading. **The introductory essay** will make the conditions more comprehensible until greater experience is gained. Junior psychiatrists and interested GPs can start to gain a knowledge of the evidence base for psychiatry, and experienced GPs will be able to use the book as a teaching aid. It is hoped that an understanding by a GP of where the psychiatrist is coming from will assist dialogue between these two professional groups.

For the psychiatrist in his professional training, the research base can only be a platform on which to build, and it will complement the necessary reading from the current professional journals. **The psychiatric interview** articles started life as my own revision for the clinical part of the MRCPsych long case and the reader approaching this examination may find the book similarly useful.

Other health and associated professionals

There is a wide variety of health professionals who may wish to gain a greater knowledge of psychiatry in a clinical format. Such people will include mental health nurses, social workers and occupationsal therapists. Psychologists will be aware of the psychological aspects, but may be interested in the other parts of psychiatry. Generally trained nurses may find the more introductory parts of this book useful.

Other professionals who may find the book of interest are those working in the non-statutory sector, but who care for people with psychiatric problems daily. For example, people working in Age Concern might still find the section on dementia (and other psychiatric illnesses that are prominent in old age) particularly helpful.

Students

Medical and nursing students may find the introductory sections helpful.

Others

It is hoped that the introductory sections will be accessible to people with no knowledge of psychiatry. Examples of people who might find the book helpful include journalists who have to report on mental health issues and lawyers who undertake medico-legal work.

1

Alcoholism

History

1. Drinking history

- Longitudinal
- Cross-Sectional.

2. Evidence of dependence

CAGE Questionnaire

- Have you felt you ought to **cut down** your drinking?
- Have people **annoyed** you by criticising your drinking?
- Have you felt **guilty** about your drinking?
- Have you ever had a first drink in the morning (**'eye-opener'**) to steady your nerves or get rid of a hangover?

Symptoms of the alcohol dependence syndrome

- Feeling of being compelled to drink
- A stereotyped pattern of drinking ('narrowing of the drinking repertoire')
- Primacy of drinking over other activities
- Altered tolerance to alcohol(initially increased tolerance; then, the patient suddenly finds that he can no longer drink like he used to, and smaller amounts get him drunk)
- Repeated withdrawal symptoms
  - nausea
  - vomiting/retching
  - tremor
  - sweating
- Relief drinking
- Reinstatement after abstinence

3. Complications

Physical

- Alimentary
  - liver damage
  - gastritis

- ❏ peptic ulcer
- ❏ oesophageal varices
- ❏ oesophageal carcinoma
- ❏ acute and chronic pancreatitis
- ◆ Hepatic
  - ❏ fatty degeneration
  - ❏ alcoholic hepatitis
  - ❏ cirrhosis
  - ❏ hepatoma
- ◆ Neurological
  - ❏ peripheral neuropathy
  - ❏ epilepsy
  - ❏ cerebellar degeneration
  - ❏ optic atrophy (rare)
  - ❏ central pontine myelinolysis (rare
  - ❏ Marchiafava-Bignami syndrome
- ◆ Head injury
- ◆ Cardiovascular
  - ❏ fatty infiltration
  - ❏ cardiomyopathy
  - ❏ hypertension
- ◆ Endocrine
  - ❏ diabetes mellitus
- ◆ Dermatological
  - ❏ rhinophyma
- ◆ Other
  - ❏ anaemia
  - ❏ proximal myopathy
  - ❏ episodic hypoglycaemia
  - ❏ haemochromatolysis
  - ❏ vitamin deficiencies
  - ❏ tuberculosis
  - ❏ gout
- ◆ Foetal alcohol syndrome

Psychological

Intoxication phenomena
- ◆ Alcoholic idiosyncratic intoxication (pathological drunkenness)
- ◆ Memory blackouts

Withdrawal phenomena
- Alcohol withdrawal syndrome
- Delirium tremens

Toxic or nutritional conditions
- Wernicke's encephalopathy
- Korsakoff's psychosis
- Alcoholic dementia

Alcohol-induced psychosis
- Alcoholic hallucinosis

Associated psychiatric disorder
- Personality deterioration
- Personality disorder
- Neurotic disorder
  - agoraphobia
  - panic disorder
  - other phobias
- Affective disorder
- Suicidal behaviour
- Impaired psychosexual function
- Pathological jealousy (morbid jealousy, Othello syndrome)

Social

- Marital and family tension
- Job losses
  - excessive days off sick
  - unemployment
  - sackings
- Road traffic accidents
- Crime
  - committed while intoxicated
  - committed to fund habit

4. Previous treatments

5. Motivation to change

Family history

- Family history of depression or alcoholism
- Violent parent(s) (often with physical or sexual abuse); absent parents

Personal history

- Truanting from school
- Drinking in gangs
- Difficulties at work: missing days as drunk (especially Monday mornings); sackings

Past medical history

- Alcohol-related illness

Past psychiatric history

- Alcohol-related disorders

Drug history

- Prescription of anti-alcohol drug
  - disulfiram
  - calcium carbonate
  - acamprosate
  - naltrexone
- Metronidazole
- Abuse of benzodiazepines

Pre-morbid personality

- Personality traits
  - people who have chronic anxiety
  - people with a pervading sense of inferiority
  - people with self-indulgent tendencies
- Interests
- Religion
- Forensic history
  - drink-related crimes
    drinking and driving, loss of car licence; violence while drunk
  - Crimes to finance alcohol
- Smoking
- Abuse of other psychoactive drugs

Social circumstances

- Job
- High risk of alcohol abuse
  - chefs, kitchen porters, barmen, brewery workers, publicans (who have easy access to alcohol)
  - executives and salesmen (who entertain on expense accounts)
  - actors and entertainers
  - journalists and printers
  - doctors
- Still in employment?
- Social support
  - still with spouse/ family?
  - professional support
    social worker; visits to alcohol treatment centre
- Housing
- Psychological support
  - AA; group therapy, etc

Psychosexual history

- Evidence of failed relationships (divorce; short term relationships); custody of children given to partner
- Alcohol abuse in the partner

Mental state examination

- Appearance
  - dishevelled
  - drunk, intoxicated, smelling of alcohol
  - ruddy nose
  - tremor
  - dirty clothes
  - clothes showing a positive view of alcohol abuse (eg 'Scrumpy Jack T-shirt') or a negative view (eg an 'AA' T-shirt)
- Behaviour
  - argumentative, aggressive, hostile
  - attempt to be polite, excessive cordiality
  - ataxic gait

- ◆ Mood and affect
  - ❐ depressed, anxious
- ◆ Speech
  - ❐ slurred
- ◆ Thoughts
  - ❐ suicidal ideation
  - ❐ paranoid ideas, jealousy
  - ❐ depressive thoughts
- ◆ Experiences
  - ❐ evidence for co-existent psychosis
- ◆ Cognition
  - ❐ evidence of impairment
- ◆ Insight
  - ❐ may be hostile to the idea that has a drinking problem

Investigations

- ◆ Blood
  - ❐ MCV
  - ❐ γGT
  - ❐ liver function tests
  - ❐ blood alcohol level
  - ❐ amylase

Management

- ◆ Education and information about safe limits and the harm caused by heavy drinking
- ◆ Assessment of the motivation to change
  - ❐ motivational interviewing
- ◆ Detoxification
  - ❐ inpatient / outpatient
  - ❐ chlordiazepoxide /(chlormethiazole)
  - ❐ vitamins B group and C
- ◆ Psychological therapies
  - ❐ group therapy
  - ❐ supportive therapy (keyworker)
  - ❐ cognitive-behavioural therapy
    relapse-prevention strategies

- ❏ family therapy
- ◆ Medication
  - ❏ anti-alcohol
    disulfiram, calcium carbimide, naltrexone, acamprosate
  - ❏ antidepressant
- ◆ Self-help groups
  - ❏ Alcoholics Anonymous; Al-Anon; Al-Ateen; Accept
- ◆ Social therapy
  - ❏ residential unit for alcoholics

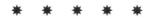

Alcohol. A bit like sex really. Or cream cakes. Naughty but nice! There is an old joke that goes around in medical circles:

Q. What is an alcoholic?

A. Someone who drinks more than his doctor.

What this really tells us is how ambivalent we are when it comes to talking about alcohol. The big mistake for a doctor talking about alcohol is not that he should avoid ambivalence — that remains inherent in talking about alcohol — but to be unaware that the moral tone often implied in such conversations is irrelevant and should be discarded. In other words, the doctor should put alcohol into its correct perspective and be clear about what the medical role really is.

The simple situation is that alcohol is a drug that acts on the central nervous system to depress its activity. In acute use, at different doses, it depresses parts of the brain selectively. Initially it affects inhibitory centres, leading to disinhibition. This is the effect that many desire, and is the reason that alcohol forms part of the fabric of many societies. However, at higher doses, it depresses other parts of the brain, making people initially maudlin, but then as it lowers the level of consciousness, it can lead to coma and even death. And even the disinhibition has its negative aspect; rather than jocularity, it can express itself in irritability and aggression, leading to fights, head injuries and broken bones; and the reduction in reaction times leads to intoxicated drivers being responsible for many road traffic accidents.

Furthermore, if it is used in high doses for extended periods of time, it causes damage to all systems of the body: cardiovascular (eg. fatty heart, high blood pressure); gut (eg. peptic ulcer, gastritis); liver (eg. cirrhosis); musculoskeletal (eg. gout); nervous (eg. epilepsy, peripheral neuropathy) and mental (alcohol dependence, anxiety disorders, depressive disorders, dementia). These are just a few examples of the many.

The apparent emphasis on the harms of alcohol should not cloud the issue: alcohol is a drug that is widely used for its pleasant effects, but has potentially serious consequences. This does not make its use right or wrong (a moral question), but one where one has to make a rational choice (a practical question).

Many people use alcohol in small quantities throughout their lives with no ill effects. They may drink two whiskies a day on coming home from work, and nothing more. They may drink on two or three days a week. A glass of wine with a meal; a couple of pints (just two) with the mates in the pub one or two nights a week; a gin and tonic at a buffet. They form the majority of society, and there is no need to change what they do. It is of little interest to the doctor.

The role of the doctor is to educate the public about how much can be drunk before there are likely to be unwanted consequences, and to detect and assist those whose drinking is excessive enough to cause them harm. This role is usually undertaken by general practitioners and public health doctors; doctors in secondary care tend to see persons who present because of alcohol-related damage that has already occurred.

It is not clear how much alcohol may be safely drunk on a regular basis, but the Royal Colleges have suggested that men can safely drink 21 units and women 14 units of alcohol in a week (not all in one go!). A unit is roughly half a pint of beer, a single measure of spirits (whisky, vodka etc.) or a glass of wine. Calculation is always rough and ready.

Psychiatrists will usually be asked to see patients when they have suffered serious physical harm from excess alcohol use (eg. a referral from a liver specialist because the patient has cirrhosis and his liver is failing) or when there is clear evidence of the alcohol dependence syndrome or social harm from alcohol, and someone (the patient, his family, his employer, the courts) has insisted that something be done about it. In these cases, the role of alcohol in the problem is obvious.

However, chronic misuse of alcohol can cause depressive illness (among other things, as mentioned earlier), and if a patient presents with depression, alcohol may not be considered as an aetiological factor, especially if there seem to be other precipitants (eg. a wife threatening to leave, recent loss of job, etc). The patient may under-report the amount of alcohol being consumed, and it is easy for the doctor to collude with the statement that the patient is a 'social drinker'. Thus, in many situations, it is necessary for the doctor to be aware that abuse of alcohol may be involved, as this is not always obvious.

Specialists identify three types of drinker. There is the 'social drinker', who drinks within limits, and who is of little concern to the doctor. This represents the majority of those who drink. Should alcohol lead to medical or social problems (eg. loss of driving licence, loss of job or relationship; stomach ulcer, etc), then the person is referred to as a 'problem drinker'. It is important to distinguish this, as many people whose use of alcohol is causing difficulties will minimise this by claiming that they are not dependent on alcohol. This may be true, but they are a group who can be helped by professionals when considering the contribution that alcohol has made to their problems. The professional can help the patient to make a choice about whether they wish to avoid or minimise the unpleasant problems by reducing the amount of alcohol consumed. As with any choice, it is the prerogative of the individual in a free society to choose a course of action that others might regard as the unwise — some people actively choose to drink themselves to death rather than give up alcohol — and it is not the role of the doctor to moralise. Attempts may be made to influence the decision of the patient by persuasion, but if the patient has the facts, then he or she can choose. The doctor should not imagine that this is necessarily a simple choice: it may be easy to see the disadvantages in continuing to drink, but for the person who has drunk to excess over many years, alcohol has some positive function in his life, and this must be addressed and dealt with before the person will be able to choose abstinence.

The third type of drinker is the 'dependent drinker'. This person has **alcohol dependence syndrome**. Any drug, acting on the brain, which is chronically administered, especially in high doses, will elicit a response that tries to minimise the effects of the drug. The number of receptors for the drug will be reduced ('down-regulation') or the receptors may adapt so that they are no longer responsive to the drug ('receptor adaptation'). As a result, if the drug is no longer there, a withdrawal syndrome will occur. Thus, a person can become physically dependent on a substance (prescribed or self-medicated). In the case of alcohol, the primary withdrawal symptoms are shaking, tremor and nausea/retching.

A doctor can detect if a person is dependent on alcohol by assessing whether they suffer from the symptoms of alcohol dependence syndrome (Edwards and Gross, 1976). The symptoms are listed in the case summary. If a person is dependent on alcohol, then if they choose to stop, it is advisable that they do so under medical supervision. Alcohol withdrawal syndrome has two potential major complications; alcohol withdrawal epileptic fits and delirium tremens, both of which can be fatal. Regimes have been developed to help people come off alcohol safely ('detoxification').

For the patient who is dependent, and also for many problem drinkers, the safer choice is to abstain from alcohol for the rest of their lives. It may be possible for problem drinkers to consider controlled drinking with professional assistance, but for the dependent drinker, a return to drinking is rarely (if ever) moderate, and abstinence must be advised.

The doctor or other health professional trying to assist the patient at this stage should be aware of the range of options available to assist the patient in abstaining; for example, Alcoholics Anonymous, day treatments and residential rehabilitation. The doctor should also recognise that it may take several attempts by the patient before he/she is successful. A relapse to drinking should not be regarded as a ' therapeutic failure', but requires further encouragement of the patient towards a plan that will be most likely to ease his/her discomfort.

✳ ✳ ✳ ✳ ✳

When assessing a patient for the possibility of an alcohol problem, the following questions need to be answered:

- does the patient use more alcohol than is healthy?
- is there evidence that the patient has developed a physical dependence on alcohol?
- what complications (physical, psychological and social) has the patient suffered from his use of alcohol?
- what are the purpose(s) for which the patient uses alcohol (pleasure, to relieve anxiety, to ward off withdrawal symptoms, etc)?
- what is the degree of motivation that the patient has to change his harmful or dependent use of alcohol?

History of presenting complaint

It is important to take both a longitudinal (history of use since the patient first drank any alcohol) and cross-sectional (current use) history of alcohol use. Although it is a commonly found clinical impression that patients underestimate their alcohol consumption, there is evidence that patient reports are less distorted than commonly assumed (Adams *et al*, 1981). The patient should be asked his age when he first drank alcohol, as an early start of alcohol use is associated with alcohol consumption and alcohol-related problems (Shuckit and Russell, 1983).

The history should reveal periods when the patient has drunk more than the recommended amounts of alcohol (in the UK the weekly limit is 21 units for men and 14 units for women). Questions should also look for evidence that the patient is dependent on alcohol. In primary care, it is sufficient to use the CAGE questionnaire (see below) as a screening tool, but in secondary care, evidence of symptoms of alcohol dependence syndrome (Edwards and Gross, 1976) should be sought. To discover this, asking the patient to describe a typical drinking day can be revealing. Tolerance is a phenomenon that has been objectively demonstrated (Lipscomb *et al*, 1980).

In those where alcohol dependence is present, there is evidence that alcoholics with onset of heavy drinking before 20 years of age have significantly more antisocial personality traits, drug abuse, bipolar disorder, panic disorder, suicide attempts and paternal alcoholism than alcoholics with onset after 20 years of age (Cadoret *et al*, 1985; Schuckit, 1985; Buydens-Branchey *et al*, 1989; Irwin *et al*, 1990). Alcoholics with onset before and after 20 years of age also differ significantly in cerebrospinal fluid concentrations of diazepam-binding inhibitor and somatostatin (Roy *et al*, 1991). Among treatment-seeking alcoholics, early age at onset is generally associated with a more severe course of alcoholism and lower cerebrospinal fluid 5-hydroxyindoleacetic acid concentration. (Fils-Aime *et al*, 1996). This forms the basis of a division of patients by Cloninger into Type I and Type II alcoholics, but the distinction between these two groups is not precise (Hall and Sannibale, 1996).

In assessment of motivation (Miller and Rollnick, 1991), the interviewer should aim to elicit:

1. The patient's perceived benefits versus harm from the present behaviour, ie. *in the patient's opinion*, do the benefits of continuing to drink outweigh the harm of continuing to drink;

2. The patient's self-acknowledged readiness to change, ie. if the patient does think that the harm of current drinking now outweighs the benefits, does the patient want to do anything to change things?

Family history

The existence of a direct genetic contribution to the aetiology of alcohol dependence has been controversial. Some recent studies have found an increased risk in monozygotic twins over dizygotic twins (Kendler *et al*, 1994; Heath *et al*, 1997; Kendler *et al*, 1997), although others have not found such a strong genetic contribution to the aetiology (Pickens *et al*, 1991).

There is an indirect genetic contribution to alcohol dependence in that the presence of a genetically determined variant of aldehyde dehydrogenase among certain races, including orientals, is associated both with a flushing reaction on consumption of alcohol and a reduced incidence of alcohol dependence (Higuchi *et al*, 1995). The suggestion that patients with alcoholism can be divided into Type I and Type II (including antisocial behaviour, parental alcoholism and parental antisocial behaviour) has been mentioned above. There is also a suggestion that the genetic contribution of alcoholism in the father may be associated with alcoholism in the male offspring, but depressive illness in the female offspring (Cadoret *et al*, 1996). Conversely, there is evidence that major depressive disorder in the parent is associated with a risk of the child developing a number of psychiatric disorders, including alcohol dependence (Weissman *et al*, 1997).

In families where there is parental psychiatric disorder, especially alcohol dependence, there is likely to be a familial environmental contribution to alcohol dependence in the patient. There is a suggestion that families whose rituals alter at a time of heavy parental drinking are most likely to show transmission of an alcohol problem to the children's generation (Wolin *et al*, 1979). There is also evidence that alcohol abuse in the parent is associated with declared child abuse and neglect (Egami *et al*, 1996).

Personal history

Fifty-nine percent of women and 30% of men in a series of alcoholic inpatients reported childhood abuse (physical and/or sexual) (Windle *et al*, 1995). Among both psychiatric patients and victims of incest found in self-help groups there is an association between childhood abuse and psychiatric disorders, such as anxiety, depression and alcohol abuse. There was a raised incidence of alcoholic fathers in these populations (Brown and Anderson, 1991; Pribor and Dinwiddie, 1992).

As well as the traits of antisocial personality disorder, there is longitudinal evidence that high novelty-seeking and low harm avoidance significantly predict early onset of substance use (eg, cigarettes, alcohol and other drugs), but reward dependence is unrelated to any of the outcomes studied among boys in kindergarten (Masse and Tremblay, 1997). Follow-up of hyperactive boys into adulthood shows a higher level of development of antisocial personality disorder (12% versus 4%) and drug abuse than controls (Mannuzza *et al*, 1998).

Past medical history

The medical history may reveal illnesses known to be associated with excessive alcohol intake, and may be the first piece of information to suggest the possibility that the patient has an alcohol problem. Alcohol abuse is associated with wide range of morbidity and with much mortality. In respect of mortality, there has consistently been found to be a J-shaped curve, in which the mortality of those who claim to drink 1–28 units of alcohol/week is actually less than those who are teetotal (eg. Doll *et al*, 1994). However, over this amount (the equivalent of two pints of beer per day), the mortality rises again above teetotal. Understanding of the basis of this phenomenon is no more than rudimentary and so it is not reasonable to advise alcohol for 'medicinal' purposes on the data currently available.

The medical complications of heavy alcohol use are numerous. A number are mentioned in the case part of this section. Reviews and discussions can be found in Paton *et al*, 1981; Lieber 1995.

Past psychiatric history

There are several mechanisms by which alcoholism and another psychiatric disorder can occur in the same individual:

- the patient suffers from alcohol abuse and another disorder that are unrelated (ie. the patient has by chance two illnesses, both psychiatric)
- there is an association of two psychiatric disorders that occurs more frequently than by chance, but it cannot be confirmed that one disorder is aetiological to the other (eg. a patient who has suffered from abuse as a child and developed both agoraphobia and alcohol dependence; alcohol abuse and bulimia nervosa [Garfinkel *et al*, 1995])
- alcohol is used in the course of another psychiatric illness that is primary (eg. a patient who drinks during an episode of hypomania; a patient who uses alcohol to ease psychotic symptoms)
- alcohol abuse directly causes the psychiatric illness (eg. anxiety disorder; Korsakoff's psychosis)
- another psychiatric disorder arises out of one of the complications of alcohol abuse (eg. post-traumatic stress disorder as a consequence of rape [Deykin and Buka, 1997]).

Sometimes the picture can be uncertain, as in the case of the relationship between alcohol and symptoms of depression. It is possible to distinguish alcohol-induced depression from a separate comorbidity of alcohol abuse and depressive illness (Schuckit *et al*, 1997). Independent episodes of depression often start before the onset of alcoholism and there may be a family history of depression. Also, there is evidence that depressed mood second to alcoholism resolves after stopping alcohol, typically within three weeks, in contrast to depressive illness with comorbid alcohol abuse (Brown *et al*, 1995).

In view of the increased incidence of suicide amongst alcoholics, risk factors have been sought. Those at greater risk of attempting suicide include: female patients; young patients or those who started drinking alcohol early; those who consume a greater amount when drinking; those with a family history of alcohol abuse or a lifetime diagnosis of additional psychiatric illness (depressive illness, substance abuse, panic disorder, phobic disorder or generalised anxiety disorder; antisocial or borderline personality disorder) (Roy *et al*, 1990; Cornelius *et al*, 1995). Completion of suicide among this group has been associated with those who continue drinking, make suicidal communication, live alone, have poor social support, are unemployed, have serious medical illness and have depressive illness (Murphy *et al*, 1992; Lesage *et al*, 1994).

Pre-morbid personality

There has been a suggestion that there is an increased incidence of personality disorder among alcoholics (Samuels *et al*, 1994), especially borderline personality disorder (Dulit *et* al, 1990), but longitudinal study suggests it may be that only antisocial personality disorder can be associated with alcoholism (Schuckit *et al*, 1994).

Religion

Religious thought and action is a coping mechanism that is inversely related to depression and associated with infrequent alcohol use in a group of medically ill old men (Koenig *et al*, 1992).

Forensic history

The presence of alcohol dependence is a risk factor among women for committing homicide (Eronen, 1995). The combination of alcohol dependence and other drug use and mental illness is a combination that represents a high risk for violence (Swartz *et al*, 1998) and the alcohol-induced psychoses and schizophrenia with alcohol abuse represents a high risk for violent criminal offences (Tiihonen *et al*, 1997). Alcoholic criminals, associated with low social status, often commit repetitive violent offences, and the risk of criminality is correlated with the severity of their own alcohol abuse (Bohman *et al*, 1982).

Social circumstances

While the family in which the alcoholic lives can be a source of support, it is not uncommon for family functioning to be disrupted. There is some evidence that during phases when the patient is stable and dry, the family can function in a flexible way, but when the patient is drinking there is a greater degree of rigidity (Steinglass, 1981). Separation and divorce are factors associated with increased anxiety, depression and alcohol abuse (Richards *et al*, 1997).

Alcohol abuse is associated with loss of family and friends. There is evidence that alcohol abusers with smaller social networks have a greater degree of psychopathology (Westermeyer and Neider, 1988). In populations of the homeless, a majority are found to have abused alcohol (eg. Susser *et al*, 1989). Alcoholics who are homeless have been found to have a high prevalence of other psychiatric disorders, more severe and more chronic drinking, with social and occupational functioning affected to a greater degree (Koegel and Burnam, 1988).

There is some evidence that those in a rural area have a higher risk of alcohol abuse or dependence than urban dwellers (Blazer *et al*, 1987).

Even accounting for the contribution of family and personal factors, there was an excess of anxiety disorder and substance use among young people who were unemployed for more than six months. There was an increase in use of: nicotine; alcohol and other substance abuse (Fergusson *et al*, 1997).

Mental state examination

The mental state examination reveals aspects of alcohol use:
- current intoxication and/or withdrawal symptoms

- evidence indicative of physical complications of alcohol abuse (if physical examination not carried out) such as rhinophyma (ruddy thickening of the nose skin)
- evidence of psychiatric complications of alcohol abuse
- aspects of current mental state that pertain specifically to alcohol abuse.

In the last category, alcoholic 'blackouts' are episodes of memory loss associated with drinking alcohol. They refer to times when the patient gives a history of alcohol use and, although appearing to others to be aware at that time, has no recall of what he/she did (Goodwin *et al*, 1969).

Prolonged alcohol abuse can cause a dementing process. However, in the early stages of treatment, cognitive impairment is often reversible. Frequently, young detoxified alcoholics do not show cognitive impairment. Cognitive impairment is more likely to be found in patients with longer lifetime consumption of alcohol, but is less likely in patients with longer abstinence (Eckardt *et al*, 1995).

Investigations

It has long been the hope that a test would be found to distinguish the alcoholic from the person who is not an alcoholic. Such a test has not appeared, and neither has a test been devised to show if the patient continues to drink, apart from the breathalyser test, which assesses levels of alcohol present at the moment of the test. Investigations, therefore, concentrate on blood and other tests of the damage that alcohol does. In particular, mean cell volume tends to be raised in chronic alcohol use and γ-glutamyl transferase is raised on acute drinking, although its interpretation is not easy (Penn and Worthington, 1983). More recently, attention has been redirected on the usefulness of carbohydrate-deficient transferrin (Schmidt *et al*, 1997).

Management

The role of the clinician is to:

- detect the presence of an alcohol problem, either by confirming it, if this is the presenting problem or , if it is not, either using a screening technique or suspecting when there are other related clues (eg. peptic ulcer)
- enhance motivation, if an alcohol problem is present, but motivation to change is not
- provide medically-supervised detoxification, if the patient is ready to do something
- provide assistance to maintain abstinence, after detoxification.

Help in these tasks can be offered by a wide variety of personnel, ranging from doctors, social workers to workers in the non-statutory sector. In addition, the medically qualified clinician can provide medication where it is indicated and can diagnose and treat medical and psychiatric complications.

If a patient is chemically-dependent on alcohol, it is generally the case that life-long abstinence is required; controlled drinking is rarely successful (Valliant, 1996).

Assessment

There is some benefit in using the CAGE questionnaire in general practice as a screening tool (King, 1986a; 1986b). More recently, the alcohol use disorders identification test has been devised for use in general practice (Piccinelli *et al*, 1997).

Treatment

A recent review of the literature on treatment of patients with alcohol problems (McCrady and Langenbucher, 1996) confirms good evidence that:

- treatment (of whatever type) is better than no treatment
- there is evidence supporting the efficacy in suitably matched patients of:
  - **brief interventions** (motivational techniques; brief skills training and advice)
  - treatments based on the psychological theory of **classical conditioning** (aversion therapies; sensitisation; cue-exposure treatment)
  - treatments based on the psychological theory of **operant conditioning** (behavioural contracting; community re-inforcement)
  - treatments based on the psychological theory of **social learning** (social skills training; cognitive therapy; relapse prevention therapy)
  - behavioural marital therapy
  - Alcoholics Anonymous.

The conclusion drawn is that long-term, low intensity treatment is most effective in the management of such patients. For the patient who is taking too much alcohol, but is not dependent, there is evidence that provision of information and education can be helpful. Assistance for the patient who is not convinced of the need to change his drinking behaviour can be provided in the form of motivational interviewing (Miller and Rollnick, 1991). A review of detoxification is provided by Hall and Zador (1997).

Maintenance of abstinence depends on how much the patient is prepared to accept. There is a variety of treatments available, for which financial constrictions add a further barrier to clinical considerations. Many patients who require detoxification will subsequently relapse, especially if the environment in which they reside is unchanged. For this reason, a number of patients benefit from a period of residential treatment: suitable patients for reputable treatment centres have a high success rate in completing the course. There are a variety of different types of courses, but programmes using the Minnesota (12-step) model, concept houses and Christian houses are most prominent.

For those unable or unwilling to go into a residential programme, day programmes can be of benefit. There is some evidence that attendance at a specialist day hospital programme may have an improved outcome in respect of alcohol use even if denial is not reduced, whereas for those who attend self-help groups, improvement in respect of drinking tends to occur more frequently when there is a corresponding reduction in denial (McKay *et al*, 1994). Alcoholics Anonymous is perhaps the best known self-help group and has some efficacy for those who are suited to the 12-step programme. Other outpatient services include relapse-prevention programmes, group therapy programmes and treatment of the family.

Drug management of alcohol abuse has always been a difficult concept, as the psychological factors predisposing to alcoholism need to be addressed if recovery is to occur and be maintained. However, medications have been used in an attempt to assist motivated people abstain from alcohol following detoxification. Early treatments were based on learning theory and involved using agents that interacted with ethanol and produced an unpleasant reaction if alcohol was consumed. On this principle, drugs such as disulfiram or calcium carbonate, which cause an unpleasant flushing reaction, have been used. There is evidence that alcohol consumption can be reduced with disulfiram use (Chick *et al*, 1992). More recently, attempts have been made to use medications that are likely to interfere with the neurobiological pathways thought to be involved in craving alcohol following detoxification, which predispose the patient to relapse. Serotonergic, opioid (Tiihonen *et al*, 1994) and gaba/ glutamatergic (Volkow *et al*, 1993; Tsai *et al*, 1995) pathways have all been thought to be involved, leading to consideration of the possible use of selective serotonin reuptake inhibitors (Kranzler *et al*, 1995), naltrexone (Volpicelli *et al*, 1992; 1995; O'Malley *et al*, 1996) and acamprosate (Sass *et al*, 1996) as accompaniments of relapse prevention programmes. The evidence of efficacy is disputed in the case of SSRIs (Kranzler *et al*, 1995). The place of medications to assist maintenance of abstinence is unclear and results are, at best, modest.

References

Adams KM, Grant I, Carlin AS, Reed R 1(981) Cross-study comparisons of self-reported alcohol consumption in four clinical groups. *Am J Psychiatry* **138**: 445–9

Blazer D, Crowell BA Jr, George LK (1987) Alcohol abuse and dependence in the rural South, *Arch Gen Psychiatry* **44**: 736–40

Bohman M, Cloninger CR, Sigvardsson S, von Knorring AL (1982) Predisposition to petty criminality in Swedish adoptees. I. Genetic and environmental heterogeneity. *Arch Gen Psychiatry* **39**: 1233–41

Brown GR, Anderson B (1991) Psychiatric morbidity in adult inpatients with childhood histories of sexual and physical abuse. *Am J Psychiatry* **148**: 55–61

Brown SA, Inaba RK, Gillin JC, Schuckit MA, Stewart MA, Irwin MR (1995) Alcoholism and affective disorder: clinical course of depressive symptoms. *Am J Psychiatry* **152**: 45–52

Buydens-Branchey L, Branchey MH, Noumair D (1989) Age of alcoholism onset. I. Relationship to psychopathology. *Arch Gen Psychiatry* **46**:225–30

Cadoret RJ, O'Gorman TW, Troughton E, Heywood E (1985) Alcoholism and antisocial personality. Interrelationships, genetic and environmental factors. *Arch Gen Psychiatry* **42**: 161–7

Cadoret RJ, Winokur G, Langbehn D, Troughton E, Yates WR, Stewart MA (1996) Depression spectrum disease, I: The role of gene-environment interaction. *Am J Psychiatry* **153**: 892–9

Chick J, Gough K, Falkowski W *et al* (1992) Disulfiram treatment of alcoholism. *Br J Psychiatry* **161**: 84

Cornelius JR, Salloum IM, Mezzich J *et al* (1995) Disproportionate suicidality in patients with comorbid major depression and alcoholism. *Am J Psychiatry* **152**: 358–64

Deykin EY, Buka SL (1997) Prevalence and risk factors for posttraumatic stress disorder among chemically dependent adolescents. *Am J Psychiatry* **154**: 752–7

Doll R, Peto R, Hall E, Wheatley K, Gray R (1994) Mortality in relation to consumption of alcohol: 13 years' observations on male British doctors. *Br Med J* **309**: 911–8

Dulit RA, Fyer MR, Haas GL, Sullivan T, Frances AJ (1990) Substance use in borderline personality disorder. *Am J Psychiatry* **147**: 1002–7

Eckardt MJ, Stapleton JM, Rawlings RR, Davis EZ, Grodin DM (1995) Neuropsychological functioning in detoxified alcoholics between 18 and 35 years of age. *Am J Psychiatry* **152**: 53–9

Edwards G, Gross MM (1976) Alcohol dependence: provisional description of a clinical syndrome. *Br Med J* I: 1058–61

Egami Y, Ford DE, Greenfield SF, Crum RM (1996) Psychiatric profile and sociodemographic characteristics of adults who report physically abusing or neglecting children. *Am J Psychiatry* **153**: 921–8

Eronen M (1995) Mental disorders and homicidal behavior in female subjects. *Am J Psychiatry* **152**: 1216–8

Fergusson DM, Horwood LJ, Lynskey MT (1997) The effects of unemployment on psychiatric illness during young adulthood. *Psychol Med* **27**: 371–81

Fils-Aime ML, Eckardt MJ, George DT, Brown GL, Mefford I, Linnoila M (1996) Early-onset alcoholics have lower cerebrospinal fluid 5-hydroxyindoleacetic acid levels than late-onset alcoholics. *Arch Gen Psychiatry* **53**: 211–6

Garfinkel PE, Lin E, Goering P *et al* (1995) Bulimia nervosa in a Canadian community sample: prevalence and comparison of subgroups. *Am J Psychiatry* **152**: 1052–8

Goodwin DW, Crane JB, Guze SB (1969) Phenomenological aspects of the alcoholic "blackout". *Br J Psychiatry* **115**: 1033–8

Hall W, Sannibale C (1996) Are there two types of alcoholism? *Lancet* **348**: 1258

Hall W, Zador D (1997) The alcohol withdrawal syndrome. *Lancet* **349**:1897–900

Heath AC, Bucholz KK, Madden PA *et al* (1997) Genetic and environmental contributions to alcohol dependence risk in a national twin sample: consistency of findings in women and men. *Psychol Med* **27**: 1381–96

Higuchi S, Matsushita S, Murayama M, Takagi S, Hayashida M (1995) Alcohol and aldehyde dehydrogenase polymorphisms and the risk for alcoholism. *Am J Psychiatry* **152**: 1219–21

Irwin M, Schuckit M, Smith TL (1990) Clinical importance of age at onset in type 1 and type 2 primary alcoholics. *Arch Gen Psychiatry* **47**: 320–24

Kendler KS, Neale MC, Heath AC, Kessler RC, Eaves LJ (1994) A twin-family study of alcoholism in women. *Am J Psychiatry* **151**: 707–15

Kendler KS, Prescott CA, Neale MC, Pedersen NL (1997) Temperance board registration for alcohol abuse in a national sample of Swedish male twins, born 1902 to 1949. *Arch Gen Psychiatry* **54**: 178–84

King M (1986a) At risk drinking among general practice attenders: validation of the CAGE questionnaire. *Psychol Med* **16**: 213–7

King MB (1986b) Case finding for at risk drinking in general practice: cost-benefit analysis. *Psychol Med* **16**: 359–63

Koegel P, Burnam MA (1988) Alcoholism among homeless adults in the inner city of Los Angeles. *Arch Gen Psychiatry* **45**: 1011–8

Koenig HG, Cohen HJ, Blazer DG *et al* (1992) Religious coping and depression among elderly, hospitalized medically ill men. *Am J Psychiatry* **149**: 1693–1700

Kranzler HR, Burleson JA, Korner P *et al* (1995) Placebo-controlled trial of fluoxetine as an adjunct to relapse prevention in alcoholics. *Am J Psychiatry* **152**: 391–7

Lesage AD, Boyer R, Grunberg F *et al* (1994) Suicide and mental disorders: a case-control study of young men. *Am J Psychiatry* **151**: 1063–8

Lieber CS (1995) Medical disorders of alcoholism. *New Eng J Med* **333**: 1058–65

Lipscomb TR, Nathan PE, Wilson GT, Abrams DB (1980) Effects of tolerance on the anxiety-reducing function of alcohol. *Arch Gen Psychiatry* **37**: 577–82

Mannuzza S, Klein RG, Bessler A, Malloy P, LaPadula M (1998) Adult psychiatric status of hyperactive boys grown up. *Am J Psychiatry 155*: 493–8

Masse LC, Tremblay RE (1997) Behavior of boys in kindergarten and the onset of substance use during adolescence. *Arch Gen Psychiatry* **54**: 62–8

McCrady BS, Langenbucher JW (1996) Alcohol treatment and health care system reform. *Arch Gen Psychiatry* **53**: 737–46

McKay JR, Alterman AI, McLellan AT, Snider EC (1994) Treatment goals, continuity of care, and outcome in a day hospital substance abuse rehabilitation program. *Am J Psychiatry* **151**: 254–9

Miller WR, Rollnick S (1991) Motivational Interviewing: Preparing People to Change Addictive Behaviour. Guilford Press, New York

Murphy GE, Wetzel RD, Robins E, McEvoy L (1992) Multiple risk factors predict suicide in alcoholism. *Arch Gen Psychiatry* **49**: 459–63

O'Malley SS, Jaffe AJ, Rode S, Rounsaville BJ (1996) Experience of a "slip" among alcoholics treated with naltrexone or placebo. *Am J Psychiatry* **153**: 281–3

Paton A, Potter JF, Saunders JB (1981) ABC of Alcohol. Detection in hospital. *Br Med J* **283**: 1594–5

Penn R, Worthington DJ (1983) Is serum γ-glutamyltransferase a misleading test? *Br Med J* **286**: 531–5

Piccinelli M, Tessari E, Bortolomasi M *et al* (1997) Efficacy of the alcohol use disorders identification test as a screening tool for hazardous alcohol intake and related disorders in primary care: a validity study. *Br Med J* **314**: 420–4

Pickens RW, Svikis DS, McGue M, Lykken DT, Heston LL, Clayton PJ (1991) Heterogeneity in the inheritance of alcoholism. A study of male and female twins. *Arch Gen Psychiatry* **48**: 19–28

Pribor EF, Dinwiddie SH (1992) Psychiatric correlates of incest in childhood. *Am J Psychiatry* **149**: 52–6

Richards M, Hardy R, Wadsworth M (1997) The effects of divorce and separation on mental health in a national UK birth cohort. *Psychol Med* **27**: 1121–8

Roy A, D, DeJong J, Moore V, Linnoila M (1990) Characteristics of alcoholics who attempt suicide. *Am J Psychiatry* **147**: 761–5

Samuels , Nestadt G, Romanoski AJ, Folstein MF, McHugh PR (1994) DSM-III personality disorders in the community. *Am J Psychiatry* **151**: 1055–62

Sass H, M, Mann K, Zieglgansberger W (1996) Relapse prevention by acamprosate. Results from a placebo-controlled study on alcohol dependence. *Arch Gen Psychiatry* **53**: 673–80

Schmidt LG, Schmidt K, Dufeu P, Ohse A, Rommelspacher H, Muller C (1997) Superiority of carbohydrate-deficient transferrin to γ-glutamyl transferase in detecting relapse in alcoholism. *Am J Psychiatry* **154**: 75–80

Schuckit MA (1985) The clinical implications of primary diagnostic groups among alcoholics. *Arch Gen Psychiatry* **42**: 1043–9

Schuckit MA, Russell JW (1983) Clinical importance of age at first drink in a group of young men. *Am J Psychiatry* **140**: 1221–3

Schuckit MA, Klein J, Twitchell G, Smith T (1994) Personality test scores as predictors of alcoholism almost a decade later. *Am J Psychiatry* **151**: 1038–42

Schuckit MA, Tipp JE, Bergman M, Reich W, Hesselbrock VM, Smith TL (1997) Comparison of induced and independent major depressive disorders in 2,945 alcoholics. *Am J Psychiatry* **154**: 948–57

Steinglass P (1981) The alcoholic family at home. Patterns of interaction in dry, wet, and transitional stages of alcoholism. *Arch Gen Psychiatry* **38**: 578–84

Susser E, Struening EL, Conover S (1989) Psychiatric problems in homeless men. Lifetime psychosis, substance use, and current distress in new arrivals at New York City shelters. *Arch Gen Psychiatry* **46**: 845–50

Swartz MS, Swanson JW, Hiday VA, Borum R, Wagner HR, Burns BJ (1998) Violence and severe mental illness: the effects of substance abuse and nonadherence to medication. *Am J Psychiatry* **155**: 226–31

Tiihonen J, Isohanni M, Rasanen P, Koiranen M, Moring J (1997) Specific major mental disorders and criminality: a 26-year prospective study of the 1966 northern Finland birth cohort. *Am J Psychiatry* **154**: 840–45

Tiihonen J, Kuikka J, Hakola P *et al* (1994) Acute ethanol-induced changes in cerebral blood flow. *Am J Psychiatry* **151**: 1505–8

Tsai G, Gastfriend DR, Coyle JT (995) The glutamatergic basis of human alcoholism. *Am J Psychiatry* **152**: 332–40

Vaillant GE (1996) A long-term follow-up of male alcohol abuse. *Arch Gen Psychiatry* **53**: 243–9

Volkow ND, Wang GJ, Hitzemann R et al (1993) Decreased cerebral response to inhibitory neurotransmission in alcoholics. *Am J Psychiatry* **150**: 417–22

Volpicelli JR, Alterman AI, Hayashida M, O'Brien CP (1992) Naltrexone in the treatment of alcohol dependence. *Arch Gen Psychiatry* **49**: 876–80

Volpicelli JR, Watson NT, King AC, Sherman CE, O'Brien CP (1995) Effect of naltrexone on alcohol "high" in alcoholics. *Am J Psychiatry* **152**: 613–5

Weissman MM, Warner V, Wickramaratne.P, Moreau D, Olfson M (1997) Offspring of depressed parents. 10 Years later. *Arch Gen Psychiatry* **54**: 932–40

Westermeyer J, Neider J (1988) Social networks and psychopathology among substance abusers. *Am J Psychiatry* **145**: 1265–9

Windle M, Windle RC, Scheidt DM, Miller GB (1995) Physical and sexual abuse and associated mental disorders among alcoholic inpatients. *Am J Psychiatry* **152**: 1322–8

Wolin SJ, Bennett LA, Noonan DL (1979) Family rituals and the recurrence of alcoholism over generations. *Am J Psychiatry* **136**(4B): 589–93

Further reading

ABC of Alcohol Series — British Medical Journal 1981–2; also available in book form, revised

American Psychiatric Association (1995) Practice guideline for the treatment of patients with substance use disorders: alcohol, cocaine. *Am J Psychiatry* **152**(11suppl): 1–80

Bissell D, Paton A, Ritson B (1982) ABC of alcohol. Help: referral. Br Med J **284**: 495–7

Lewis KO, Paton A (1981) ABC of alcohol. Tools of detection. *Br Med J* **283**: 1531–2

Paton A, Saunders JB (1981) ABC of alcohol. Definitions. *Br Med J* **283**: 1248–50

Paton A, Potter JF, Saunders JB (1981) ABC of Alcohol. Nature of the problem. *Br Med J* **283**: 1318–9

Paton A, Saunders JB (1981) ABC of alcohol. Asking the right questions. *Br Med J* **283**:1248–50

Paton A, Potter JF, Saunders JB (1981) ABC of alcohol. Detection in hospital. *Br Med J* **283**: 1594–5

Ritson B (1982) ABC of alcohol. Helping the problem drinker. Br Med J **284**: 327–9

Ritson B (1982) ABC of alcohol. Help: drugs. Br Med J **284**: 399

Saunders JB, Paton A (1981) ABC of alcohol. Alcohol in the body. *Br Med J* **283**: 1380–1

Smerdon G, Paton A (1982) ABC of alcohol. Detection in general practice. *Br Med J* **284**: 255–7

2

Anorexia nervosa

History

1. Symptoms of anorexia

History of anorexia

- Amount of weight lost, maximum and minimum weight, body mass index fluctuation
- Methods of keeping down weight
  - exercise
  - laxatives, diuretics, thyroxine, insulin (in diabetes)
  - vomiting
- Amenorrhoea

Anorectic attitudes

- Preoccupation with body image
  - distorted, perceived as being too fat
  - cheeks, breasts, thighs, buttocks, abdomen
- Preoccupation with food
  - concern that eating too much
  - rumination

    food is bad; calorific value of food; what to select; how to get rid of it; preoccupation in cooking for others
  - hiding, eating alone, food fads

Other concerns about life

- Leaving home
- Sexual relationships
- Parental dysharmony
- Responsibilities of adulthood
- Sexual abuse

2. Complications

Psychological

- Bulimic episodes
- Depression

- ◆ Obsessional thoughts
  - ❏ food, washing, dressing, tidiness
- ◆ Alcohol abuse (multi-impulsive)
- ◆ Stealing
- ◆ Deliberate self-harm
- ◆ Schizophrenia (rare).

Physical

- ◆ Malnutrition
  - ❏ wasting and proximal weakness of limbs
  - ❏ cold peripheries
  - ❏ chilblains
  - ❏ lanugo
  - ❏ bradycardia
  - ❏ hypotension
  - ❏ ankle oedema
- ◆ Secondary sexual characteristics preserved
- ◆ Osteoporosis, pathological fractures.

Family history

- ◆ Profession of father (higher socioeconomic class)
- ◆ Obese mother
- ◆ High parental expectations
- ◆ Parental discord
- ◆ Loss of a parent through death or divorce
- ◆ Family history (runs in families).

Personal history

- ◆ High achievement at school/university
- ◆ Occupations associated with eating disorders
  - ❏ ballet

Past medical history

- ◆ Diabetes mellitus

Past psychiatric history

- Previous obesity (rare)
- Episodes of deliberate self-harm
- Past history of treatment at slimming clinics
- Previous episodes of psychosis
  - ❏ induced by amphetamine-like slimming pill
  - ❏ re-feeding psychosis.

Drug history

- Amphetamines prescribed as slimming pills
- Diuretics
- Laxatives.

Pre-morbid personality

- Competitiveness
- Quiet, compliant, overcontrolled
- Alcohol abuse, abuse of illicit drugs.

Psychosexual history

- Onset of menstruation (if at all)
  - ❏ secondary amenorrhoea
- Number of sexual partners (if at all)
- Ambivalence about sexual orientation

Social circumstances

- Job
  - ❏ involved with food (eg. Chef)
  - ❏ ballet dancer
  - ❏ actress
  - ❏ athlete
- May be living with parents.

Physical examination

- Weight; height; body mass index (W/H², where W = weight in kilograms and H = height in metres)
- Need to rule out a primary organic syndrome
- Evidence of inadequate nutrition/physiology of starvation
  - ☐ difficulty rising from a squatting position (proximal myopathy)
  - ☐ bradycardia
  - ☐ acrocyanosis
  - ☐ hypotension
  - ☐ anaemia
- Evidence of self-induced vomiting
  - ☐ pitting of the nails (secondary to repeated induction of vomiting)
  - ☐ calluses on the dorsum of hand (Russell's sign)
  - ☐ dental caries
  - ☐ parotid enlargement ('hamster appearance')
- Lanugo hair
- Emaciation
- Loss of secondary sexual characteristics

Physical investigations

- Blood
  - ☐ anaemia; normal ESR; cyclical neutropenia with relative lymphocytosis
  - ☐ hypokalaemic alkalosis
  - ☐ hypercholesterolaemia
  - ☐ hypercarotenaemia
  - ☐ reduced levels of copper, zinc and magnesium
  - ☐ liver function tests
  - ☐ blood tests associated with osteoporosis
  - ☐ functional hypothyroidism
  - ☐ reduced fat soluble vitamins
- Cardiological
  - ☐ ECG
- Neurophysiological
  - ☐ EEG
  - ☐ generalised slowing of dominant frequency
- Radiological
  - ☐ PA and lateral chest X-ray; skull X-ray

- ❏ ovarian ultrasound
- ❏ CT scan
  cortical atrophy, ventricular enlargement, cerebellar atrophy
- ◆ Dental examination.

Mental state examination

- ◆ Baggy clothing
- ◆ Self-cutting (usually in areas hidden by clothes)
- ◆ Tendency to split staff
- ◆ Angry affect; sense of attempt to control interview
- ◆ Denial of illness
- ◆ Unwillingness to co-operate with treatment.

Management

- ◆ Medical admission if severely cachectic
- ◆ Psychiatric inpatient admission
  - ❏ contract with patient
  - ❏ refeeding
    target weight; bed rest; supervised eating; prevent vomiting/purgation; privileges withdrawn
- ■ getting up, dressing, time off ward, visitors
  - ❏ pharmacological treatment
    Neuroleptics; antidepressant treatment
  - ❏ individual psychotherapy
  - ❏ group therapy
  - ❏ family therapy
  - ❏ assertiveness training
  - ❏ art therapy
  - ❏ relaxation exercises
  - ❏ stress management
- ◆ psychiatric outpatient management
  - ❏ return responsibility to the patient (not their carers)
    support relatives
  - ❏ slow weight gain
    regular weighing, structured re-feeding, dietary advice
  - ❏ motivate by blunt realities

- ☐ family therapy
- ☐ social intervention
  independent accommodation and support
- ☐ social skills training
- ☐ day hospital
- ☐ self-help books
- ☐ self-help groups (eg. Eating Disorders Association).

In chronic patients, paradoxing the patients occasionally helps, ie. suggest to the patient that it may be better to keep the anorexia.

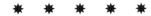

The scene is repeated all around the world, in every country and land; the cries of exasperated mothers, desperately trying to persuade their young children to eat. In the developed world, it is aggravated by the existence of fast and processed food. It seems that whatever a mother does, the child only seems to want to eat what the mother thinks is rubbish. Chocolate, chips, sweets... Will the child ever grow properly?

Perhaps you are a parent and this scenario is only too familiar. Or your friends or relatives have small children and you see what they go through trying to get their precious ones to eat. Parents handle the situation in different ways. Some are tolerant and let the children eat what and when they want; others seek the advice of specialists, either professionals or the magazines and journals. However it is approached, feeding the young is a major concern and, for some parents, mealtimes are the scene of a protracted and daily battle of wills with their children.

Look in the newspapers and magazines. Pictures stare out at you, thrust into your face. These are the people in the limelight, the famous (and rich?). They are the successful ones. Don't you just want to be like them? You can (the papers go on), if you want to. If you really want to. If you're **hungry** enough for it. Success, riches and fame can be yours. But only if you are one of the beautiful people. Only if you look right. Pretty face. Beautiful clothes by the best designers. Make-up with the latest scientific discoveries that is 'kind to your skin'. And **thin** . . .

The two scenarios above are the background, not the cause to problems that some people, in particular adolescent women, have with eating. Eating disorders are not common, but concerns about food are. They are talked about all the time. So is weight. It is true that to be overweight increases the risk of dying from diseases, such as heart disease. But it is also true that there is a higher risk of dying from being underweight, but this is a less frequent subject for discussion.

Adolescence is a difficult time. The person is starting to develop her own opinions and beliefs, not just agreeing with those of her parents. She is trying to find her place in the world. What will she do with her life? Will it be worthwhile (and will she be worthwhile)?

Will she be the same as every other woman, a 'downtrodden' wife and mother? Or will she make her own mark in the world? Will she be **special**?

Many people go through the years of adolescence with relatively little trauma. They start working, take on adult responsibilities and realise that they are no different from others — and are pleased that this is the case. They become worthwhile members of society by being members of society.

But for a few, this transition is not as straightforward. External features, such as looks, matter above everything. Persuading adults to respect them is difficult, and they may come to feel that the only way to gain the esteem of others is to be **the best**. If you are better than others, then you cannot be worthless or useless. And you have to show that you are better. They have to know it. But what can you do better than others? You do not yet have the skills to become — and remain — a world-famous person (there are a few exceptions to this). And what is it that parents and your peers are all talking about? **Food, weight and dieting**. There it is. You have it. You can show that you are a better person than your friend by dieting better than her, by showing that you are more in control of your urges to eat than she is. You miss a few meals — people don't notice. You lose a bit of weight and you are proud of yourself. You lose more weight than your friend and you are ecstatic. But it is not so easy to keep it from others, so you have to make sure that they do not know. You stop eating with the family — maybe they are too busy to notice. You are hungry (but are 'beating' it); but now and again you put on weight. You make sure that you only eat foods with few calories in them, like salads. You find out that you can get rid of body weight by getting rid of body water. There are drugs called diuretics that help you do this. You find out that you can lower your weight by the use of laxatives. And there are drugs that stop you feeling hungry.

At some stage, someone starts to notice. Depending on how you are holding up, it is easier or harder to keep it hidden. Your parents, typically your mother, may have been colluding with you. Your choice of baggy jumpers and leggings is your way of showing your own choice in clothing. But eventually something happens and it is all out in the open. You are at the doctor's and he/she (the doctor) is saying that you have got **anorexia nervosa**! Your success, your pride and joy, your whole being in the world is no more than an illness? And a mental illness at that! No way!

The description is a bit dramatised and the processes that lead this way are all unconscious, but this is often how anorexia nervosa develops. It is a disorder in which the patient is desperate to lose weight, even though she is starving. The only way she can feel of value is to diet and lose weight. If you stop her doing this, what will be left of her?

As a result, the patient resists the diagnosis and fiercely resists attempts to stop her dieting. Her parents despair. The doctor is very concerned for her well-being, as her lack of nutrition makes her physically very ill, with death a real possibility. Her parents and the doctors try to force her to eat. It becomes a battle of wills and, if not handled carefully, it can become a duel literally to the death.

Understanding of this process allows a way forward in treatment. At the time of diagnosis, the professionals wishing to help the girl who is anorexic need to guide her towards putting on enough weight and eating enough to be safe, but at the same time must avoid trampling on her fragile self-esteem. The patient should be recognised as a person, who needs to be helped to make her own decision to put on weight. Initially, the patient will need a firm, but gentle hand. As crises occur, she may slip back and lose weight, so the process of weight gain may take weeks or months. While this is happening, arrangements should be made for psychotherapy at various levels to help her develop the self-esteem and value that she has never had. In the beginning, it may be the support of her anorexic peer group in a day hospital that allows her to question her attitudes; a sympathetic therapist may be able to help her look at her distorted view of her body; the family may be seen in treatment, to help it look at the underlying beliefs and interactions that might, unwittingly, have contributed to the patient developing and maintaining anorexia nervosa. Later on it may be possible to carry out some more detailed psychotherapy with her on her own.

For some patients whose body weight is so low that it is life threatening, it may be necessary to admit them to hospital to enforce feeding. It may be necessary to continue this until her weight is such that treatment can be started to help the patient recover from the disorder. Such a step should only be taken when other avenues have been exhausted. But for those who can stay in treatment, many will improve. Over time, more mature and positive ways of thinking can develop and weight can be regained and remain steady.

✹　✹　✹　✹　✹

History of presenting complaint

In the assessment of a patient with an eating disorder, the points of assessment are:

1. Does the person have a formal eating disorder that would be diagnosable by a psychiatric classification (anorexia nervosa [± bulimic symptoms]; bulimia nervosa; or morbid obesity);

2. If so, are there any physical and/or psychiatric complications that the patient is suffering from and which need to be addressed;

3. Are there any underlying psychological issues that are perpetuating the illness?

This section deals only with anorexia nervosa.

It is important to distinguish anorexia (loss of appetite) or other symptoms related to the gastrointestinal tract with the psychiatric disorder **anorexia nervosa**. Patients with advanced cancer, or many chronic physical illnesses feel unwell and lose their appetite as a result. This is not a psychiatric disorder. In anorexia nervosa, patients do not lose their appetite: indeed they are starving. For the patient with anorexia nervosa, the underlying perception is that she is fat, looks terrible and the only way that she can improve the situation is to lose weight. This she can only do by not taking in more calories or weight-inducing substances (including water) and by getting rid of as many calories or weight-inducing substances as possible. Far from having no appetite, the patient is constantly thinking about food, and preparing it for others (who show the patient that they do not have the patient's strength of character by eating the food). It is these beliefs (referred to as **anorectic attitudes**) together with perfectionism and cognitive restraint (Sullivan *et* al, 1998) that characterise anorexia nervosa as a psychological disorder. Thus, in making the diagnosis, the clinician should look not only for the triplet of anorexia, method of weight loss and amenorrhoea, but also establish that the weight loss is accompanied by anorectic attitudes.

The longitudinal history of the illness may include a prodromal phase in the months and years before presentation in which there may be precipitating events resulting in loss of self-esteem and increased consciousness of physical appearance. This may be followed by the development of anorectic attitudes, and include an unreasonable fear of eating and a pride in the ability to lose weight. Finally, the severity of the starvation forces the patient to accept that she is ill (Casper and Davis, 1977). In the year prior to the development of the illness, many patients with anorexia nervosa have problems, especially of life stresses with family and friends or with sexuality (Schmidt *et al* 1997).

The role of amenorrhoea as a diagnostic symptom has recently been questioned. While there is no dispute that it is very common in patients with anorexia nervosa, a number of patients can be diagnosed as having the disorder by DSM-III-R standards who do not have amenorrhoea as a symptom, and this has been referred to as a partial syndrome of anorexia nervosa (Garfinkel *et al*, 1996). This view (developed through clinical experience) implies that weight loss is a primary phenomenon and examination of symptomatology over time (four year follow-up of adolescents), has led some researchers to consider the eating disorders of anorexia nervosa and bulimia nervosa to be part of an eating disorders spectrum (van der Ham *et al*, 1997).

The amount of weight loss has prognostic significance, with the majority of those who died in a nine and a half year follow up study having a body mass index (BMI; weight in kg divided by height in metres squared; $W(kg)/H(m)^2$) less than $13kg/m^2$ at presentation (Hebebrand *et al*, 1997).

Family history

There is some genetic vulnerability, with some studies reporting a concordance rate of around 50% for monozygotic twins and 10% for dizygotic twins, and first-degree female relatives of patients have a higher risk of developing the disorder than controls (Garner, 1993). While there is evidence to support a genetic contribution to dieting behaviour, drives for thinness, body dissatisfaction and body mass index, there is little support for the suggestion that the family environment contributes to this picture (Garfinkel *et al*, 1983; Rutherford *et al*, 1993).

There has been an impression that anorexia nervosa is more common in families of a higher social class, but it would appear that this arises from studies in hospital-based populations. Studies in less specialist setting (such as surveys of schoolgirls) suggest that the disorder is represented across the social classes (Patton *et al*, 1990; Garner, 1993) Similarly, sibling position is thought by some to be less important than previously suggested (Patton *et al*, 1990; Garner, 1993).

Patients with a diagnosis of anorexia nervosa give a history of parental depression, parental treatment for emotional disorder/drug dependency, parental serious disharmony and serious sexual abuse more frequently than controls (Garfinkel *et al*, 1996).

It is important to consider the relationship with parents, as poor family relationships have been suggested as a poor prognostic factor (Rosenvinge and Mouland, 1990). Descriptions of the family have included descriptions of mothers as dominant, intrusive and ambivalent, and fathers as passive and ineffectual. Patterns of interaction described as enmeshment, overprotectiveness, rigidity and family conflict avoidance have also been identified (Garner, 1993), and seem to have some specificity for anorexia nervosa, unlike high expressed emotion, which may be present in families under stress from other conditions (Blair *et al*, 1995). However, the presence of high parental expressed emotion has been found to contribute to patients dropping out of treatment (Szmukler *et al*, 1985). It is also important to be aware that many patients with anorexia nervosa profess to be happy with their families (Heron and Leheup, 1984).

The evidence suggests some genetic overlap between anorexia nervosa and bulimia nervosa, but there is no overlap with major depressive disorder, obsessive-compulsive disorder, and substance dependence, although obsessional personality trait may be a familial risk factor for anorexia nervosa (Lilenfeld *et al*, 1998).

Personal history

A history of sexual abuse has been found frequently in patients with eating disorders. However, it would appear that for this group of patients, the abuse serves as a vulnerability factor for psychiatric disorder in general rather than specifically for an eating disorder (Vize and Cooper, 1995). It appears that not only childhood adversity, but aspects of the child's response to such adversity affects whether the patient will go on to develop an eating disorder. Childhood helplessness and a lack of childhood mastery have been identified as more prominent in patients with eating disorders (Troop and Treasure, 1997).

In adolescence, there is some evidence that social class, drug use and indicators of 'the model child' (high grades, high occupational aspirations and much homework) are not related to eating problems. However, obesity, early puberty, low self-esteem, depression, unstable self-perception, with body dissatisfaction and adoption of idols with perfect bodies, and alcohol intoxication do seem to be related (Wichstrom, 1995). Patients with anorexia nervosa show delay in all sexual milestones (age of first kiss, masturbation, genital fondling and age of first intercourse (Schmidt *et al*, 1995).

There is evidence that anorexia nervosa is more common in certain professions, such as gymnastics, figure skating, ballet and modelling (Garner and Garfinkel, 1980; Garner 1993). There seems to be an association between competitiveness in the environment and the likelihood of developing anorexia nervosa (Garner and Garfinkel, 1980). Exercising is often used as a mechanism for inducing weight loss. However, there is a suggestion that many patients with anorexia nervosa have a history of exercising and taking part in sports, such as competitive athletics prior to onset of the disorder (Davis *et al*, 1994).

Past medical history

The presentation of anorexia nervosa has been reported as being secondary to organic disorder, such as hypothalamic tumour (Heron and Johnston, 1976; White *et al*, 1977;

Weller and Weller, 1982), but this is rare. Occasionally, medical illnesses, such as trauma (road traffic accident [Damlouji and Ferguson, 1985]) or viral illness (Park *et al*, 1995) have been suggested as precipitants of anorexia nervosa. Medical illnesses, such as diabetes mellitus, have also shown an association with abnormal eating attitudes (Steel *et al*, 1989).

There have been reports of anorexia nervosa in patients with various chromosomal abnormalities, including: Turner's syndrome (Fieldsend, 1988), XY gonadal dysgenesis (McCluskey and Lacey, 1992) and possibly Klinefelter's syndrome (Hindler and Norris, 1986). It would seem that people with anorexia nervosa are more likely to have past history of one or more medical illnesses. It has been suggested that this may be a risk factor, perhaps through the mechanism of family enmeshment and overprotection operating at the time of the illness. Evidence suggests that physical illness is not a precipitant of anorexia, nor is there an excess of illnesses of the alimentary tract (Patton *et al*, 1986). Surprisingly, in view of the importance of body image in the development of anorexia nervosa, there have been reports of anorexia nervosa in patients blind since birth (Touyz *et al*, 1988) and in others blind since the age of two years (Yager *et al*, 1986).

Past psychiatric history

Evidence suggests that patients with anorexia show much psychiatric comorbidity, for example, with general anxiety disorder and simple phobia (Garfinkel *et al*, 1996). Association with depression is much harder to identify, as it has recently been recognised that low mood is a consequence of starvation and, for many patients, mood improves as re-feeding brings the patient closer to normal weight. There is an association with personality disturbances, but with many studies of personality carried out on patients with established disease, the direction of causality is not certain (Garner, 1993). There is also comorbidity with obsessional-compulsive disorder (Thiel *et al*, 1995), anxiety disorders and alcohol (Sullivan *et al*, 1998) and drug abuse (Braun *et al*, 1994).

Major psychological stressors that lead to psychiatric disorder have been reported as precipitating anorexia nervosa. These include termination of pregnancy (Thomas and Harris, 1982) and torture (Fahy *et al*, 1988).

It is clear from early research that anorexia nervosa and bulimia nervosa are distinct conditions (Garfinkel *et al* 1980). However, patients with anorexia nervosa do have episodes of bingeing.

Drug history

It is important to enquire about medications, such as diuretics, purgatives and thyroid hormones that are being used to precipitate weight loss. It should be borne in mind that these medications may be fatal, for example, ipecac (Friedman, 1984; Romig, 1984).

Pre-morbid personality

It has been found that patients with eating disorders have an increased likelihood of diagnoses of schizotypal, borderline and avoidant personality disorders compared to those with other psychiatric diagnoses (Oldham *et al*, 1995). No difference has been found between anorexia nervosa and bulimia nervosa personality disorder diagnoses (Gartner *et al*, 1989). In anorexic patients, it has been suggested that those who diet are more often intense, introverted, socially withdrawn individuals, whereas those who vomit tend to be more outgoing (Beumont *et al*, 1976). Patients with anorexia nervosa often drink beverages containing caffeine (coffee, diet cola) that suppress the appetite while containing few calories (Sours 1983).

Social history

Living in cities is a factor in bulimia nervosa, but not anorexia nervosa, for which there is no difference between rural and urban incidence rates (Hoek *et al*, 1995).

Psychosexual history

For many patients, sexual development is unclear. A number of male patients with anorexia nervosa class themselves as asexual (Carlat *et al*, 1997). Some women with anorexia nervosa feel sexually inhibited and that sexual challenge precipitated their illness. They also report a decrease in sexual interest and enjoyment following weight loss; the effect on actual sexual behaviour is variable, with some showing increased and others decreased sexual behaviour when ill (Beumont *et al*, 1981).

Mental state

Mood state

It is important to try to distinguish between depressive illness and low mood induced by metabolic starvation. There is evidence that some anorexic patients with symptoms of low mood respond to treatment of their food disorder (Wamboldt *et al*, 1987).

Perfectionism

Patients with anorexia nervosa show a need for perfectionism, order and precision, even when well (Srinivasagam *et al*, 1995).

Body image

Overestimation of body size occurs in normal adolescents (Strober *et al*, 1979) and in pregnant women (Slade 1977), as well as in many (but not all) patients with anorexia nervosa. However, the distortion persists in patients with anorexia nervosa compared to normal university students (Horne *et al*, 1991). The abnormal estimate of body size by patients with anorexia nervosa persists after weight gain (Garfinkel *et al*, 1979) and the degree of overestimation is related to the risk of relapse (Button *et al*, 1977). Compared with normal adolescents, patients with anorexia nervosa are described as showing greater prevalence of experiences denoting estrangement from the body, insensitivity to body sensations and weakness of body boundaries (Strober *et al*, 1979). Patients with anorexia nervosa respond to a greater degree than comparison women in overestimation of women with 'idealised' bodies portrayed in the media (Hamilton and Waller, 1993).

Psychosis

Very occasionally, patients with anorexia nervosa can experience a transient psychosis. The features are not always consistent with a picture of schizophrenia or hypomania, nor are they clearly 'organic'. Explanation of these psychoses is uncertain, but it has been thought that there might be a 're-feeding' psychosis, in which the process of re-feeding the patient causes psychosis (Grounds, 1982).

Cognitive function

When ill, patients with anorexia nervosa have difficulties with tasks that measure attention (eg. symbol digit test), visuospatial ability and memory. Patients with lower weight perform less ably in these tests. This poor performance is associated with enlargement of lateral ventricles, dilated cortical and cerebellar sulci measured on CT scan and MRI (Palazidou *et al*, 1990; Kingston *et al*, 1996). Tissue loss is reversible with re-feeding (Swayze *et al*, 1996).

Physical examination

Although there are physical changes that are the result of the disorder, many physical, and sometimes life-threatening, conditions are the result of starvation rather than the underlying pathology. Physical changes resulting from the disorder include marked weight loss, pitting of the nails of fingers used to induce vomiting and parotid enlargement as a result of frequent vomiting (Gunther, 1988). The main physical complications of anorexia nervosa include:

- cardiovascular complications, particularly those due to electrolyte disturbances
- haematologic changes (Alloway *et al*, 1988)
- electrolyte disturbances (particularly from vomiting, diuretic and laxative abuse)
  - ❖ hypokalaemia: rare in outpatients (Greenfeld *et al*, 1995)
  - ❖ hypoglycaemia (Ratcliffe and Bevan, 1985)
  - ❖ metabolic alkalosis (Warren and Steinberg, 1979)
  - ❖ low serum albumin (Herzog *et al*, 1997)
  - ❖ low serum cholesterol (Bhanji and Mattingly, 1981)
  - ❖ low serum carotene (Bhanji and Mattingly 1981)
- osteoporosis, which may present with bone or back pain and pathological fracture (Brotman and Stern, 1985). The average spinal, radial, and femoral bone mineral density in anorexic women is lower than in normal control subjects (Salisbury and

Mitchell, 1991).Osteoporosis is not necessarily related to under nutrition and although in some patients osteoporosis is reversed by administration of oestrogen, it is not the case in all patients (Mehler, 1997).

- neurological (Byrne *et al*, 1993) and neuromuscular complications (Alloway *et al*, 1988)
- renal disease (Herzog *et al*, 1997).

A discussion of the electrolyte abnormalities, cardiac complications, abnormal glucose and bone metabolism can be found in the reviews of Beumont *et al* (1993) and Sharp and Freeman (1993). It is also important to be aware of the dangers of rapid intravenous hyperalimentation (Sharp and Freeman, 1993), with the possibility of precipitation of heart failure in the course of re-feeding (Powers, 1982). Herzog *et al* (1997) followed up a group of patients for 12 years and found:

- low serum albumin ($\leq$ 36g/l) and body weight $\leq$ 60% average at presentation predict lethal course
- high serum creatinine and uric acid predict chronic course
- these findings were initially reversible with normal food intake.

It would appear that the major contribution to mortality in patients with anorexia nervosa are these complications and suicide (Crisp *et al*, 1992).

Management

The principles of management involve:

- ensuring weight gain to normal levels (BMI 20–25 in adult women) and reducing behaviours designed to cause weight loss
- treating physical and psychological complications of the disorder
- addressing the psychological aspects of the disorder.

In encouraging the patient to accept weight gain, it is useful to provide feedback of how she is progressing. Weighing three times weekly is sufficient for this purpose (Touyz *et al*, 1990). Good prognostic indicators for weight gain include less denial of illness, less psychosexual immaturity and admitting to feeling hunger (Halmi *et al*, 1979). It should be borne in mind that as weight is gained, kinetic energy used increases (Falk *et al*, 1985) and, in patients discharged from hospital before reaching normal weight, there is a higher incidence of re-hospitalisation in the succeeding two years (Baran *et al*, 1995). There is some evidence to suggest that after reaching normal weight, patients with anorexia have an increased caloric requirement for maintaining weight (Weltzin *et al*, 1991). Resumption of menses occurs at 90% of standard body weight, two kg above the weight at which menses ceased. Over 80% of patients resume menstruation within six months of reaching these weights (Golden *et al*, 1997).

Drug treatment seems to play little part in the treatment of anorexia nervosa. Fluoxetine (Attia *et al*, 1998), cyproheptadine (Halmi *et al*, 1986) and sulpiride (Vandereycken, 1984) have not been shown to provide any significant clinical benefit.

Psychological approaches are the mainstay of treatment. In the short-term, for weight gain in severely thin patients, behaviour modification has been used to assist re-feeding (Halmi *et al*, 1975), but even when patients have reached the recommended weight, full recovery requires psychological change in respect of anorectic attitudes (Windauer *et al*, 1993). Body image therapy has been tried.

In the longer term, individual and family therapy have been helpful at one year (Crisp *et al,* 1991) and five years (Eisler *et al*, 1997), although much of the improvement can be attributed to the natural history of the disorder. Family therapy is more helpful in younger patients (Russell *et al*, 1987).

References

Alloway R, Shur E, Obrecht R, Russell GF (1988) Physical complications in anorexia nervosa. Haematological and neuromuscular changes in 12 patients. *Br J Psychiatry* **153**: 72–5

Attia E, Haiman C, Walsh BT, Flater SR (1998) Does fluoxetine augment the inpatient treatment of anorexia nervosa? *Am J Psychiatry* **155**: 548–51

Baran SA, Weltzin TE, Kaye WH (1995) Low discharge weight and outcome in anorexia nervosa. *Am J Psychiatry* **152**: 1070–72

Beumont PJ, George GC, Smart DE (1976) 'Dieters' and 'vomiters and purgers' in anorexia nervosa. *Psychol Med* **6**: 617–22

Beumont PJ, Abraham SF, Simson KG (1981) The psychosexual histories of adolescent girls and young women with anorexia nervosa. *Psychol Med* **11**: 131–40

Beumont PJV, Russell JD, Touyz SW (1993) Treatment of anorexia nervosa. *Lancet* **341**: 1635–40

Bhanji S, Mattingly D (1981) Anorexia nervosa: some observations on "dieters" and "vomiters", cholesterol and carotene. *Br J Psychiatry* **139**: 238–41

Blair C, Freeman C, Cull A (1995) The families of anorexia nervosa and cystic fibrosis patients. *Psychol Med* **25**: 985–93

Braun DL, Sunday SR, Halmi KA (1994) Psychiatric comorbidity in patients with eating disorders. *Psychol Med* **24**: 859–67

Brotman AW, Stern TA (1985) Osteoporosis and pathologic fractures in anorexia nervosa. *Am J Psychiatry* **142**: 495–6

Button EJ, Fransella F, Slade PD (1977) A reappraisal of body perception disturbance in anorexia nervosa. *Psychol Med* **7**: 235–43

Byrne A, Byrne M, Hnatko G, Zibin T (1993) Neurological complications of anorexia nervosa. *Br J Psychiatry* **163**: 418–9

Carlat DJ, Camargo CA Jr, Herzog DB (1997) Eating disorders in males: a report on 135 patients. *Am J Psychiatry* **154**: 1127–32

Casper RC, Davis JM (1977) On the course of anorexia nervosa. *Am J Psychiatry* **134**: 974–8

Crisp AH, Norton K, Gowers S *et al* (1991) A controlled study of the effect of therapies aimed at adolescent and family psychopathology in anorexia nervosa. *Br J Psychiatry* **159**: 325–33

Crisp AH, Callender JS, Halek C, Hsu LK (1992) Long-term mortality in anorexia nervosa. A 20-year follow-up of the St George's and Aberdeen cohorts. *Br J Psychiatry* **161**: 104–7

Damlouji NF, Ferguson JM (1985) Three cases of posttraumatic anorexia nervosa. *Am J Psychiatry* **142**: 362–3

Davis C, Kennedy SH, Ravelski E, Dionne M (1994) The role of physical activity in the development and maintenance of eating disorders. *Psychol Med* **24**: 957–67

Eisler I, Dare C, Russell GF, Szmukler G, le Grange D, Dodge E (1997) Family and individual therapy in anorexia nervosa. A 5-year follow-up. *Arch Gen Psychiatry* **54**: 1025–30

Fahy TA, Robinson PH, Russell GF, Sheinman B (1988) Anorexia nervosa following torture in a young African woman. *Br J Psychiatry* **153**: 385–7

Falk JR, Halmi KA, Tryon WW (1985) Activity measures in anorexia nervosa. *Arch Gen Psychiatry* **42**: 811–14

Fieldsend B (1988) Anorexia nervosa and Turner's syndrome. *Br J Psychiatry* **152**: 270–71

Garfinkel PE, Moldofsky H, Garner DM (1979) The stability of perceptual disturbances in anorexia nervosa. *Psychol Med* **9**: 703–8

Garfinkel PE, Moldofsky H, Garner DM (1980) The heterogeneity of anorexia nervosa. Bulimia as a distinct subgroup. *Arch Gen Psychiatry* **37**: 1036–40

Garfinkel PE, Garner DM, Rose J *et al* (1983) A comparison of characteristics in the families of patients with anorexia nervosa and normal controls. *Psychol Med* **13**: 821–8

Garfinkel PG, Goering ELP, Spegg C *et al* (1996) Should amenorrhoea be necessary for the diagnosis of anorexia nervosa? *Br J Psychiatry* **168**: 500–6

Garner DM, Garfinkel PE (1980) Socio-cultural factors in the development of anorexia nervosa. *Psychol Med* **10**: 647–56

Garner DM (1993) Pathogenesis of anorexia nervosa. *Lancet* **341**: 1631–5

Gartner AF, Marcus RN, Halmi K, Loranger AW (1989) DSM-III-R personality disorders in patients with eating disorders. *Am J Psychiatry* **146**: 1585–91

Golden NH, Jacobson MS, Schebendach J, Solanto MV, Hertz SM, Shenker R (1997) Resumption of menses in anorexia nervosa. *Arch Ped Adolesc Med* **151**: 16–21

Greenfeld D, Mickley D, Quinlan DM, Roloff P (1995) Hypokalemia in outpatients with eating disorders. *Am J Psychiatry* **152**: 60–3

Grounds A (1982) Transient psychoses in anorexia nervosa: a report of 7 cases. *Psychol Med* **12**: 107–13

Gunther R (1988) Anorexia nervosa and parotid enlargement. *Am J Psychiatry* **145**: 650

Halmi KA, Powers P, Cunningham S (1975) Treatment of anorexia nervosa with modification. Effectiveness of formula feeding and isolation. *Arch Gen Psychiatry* **32**: 93–6

Halmi KA, Goldberg SC, Casper RC, Eckert ED, Davis JM (1979) Pretreatment predictors of outcome in anorexia nervosa. *Br J Psychiatry* **134**: 71–8

Halmi KA, Eckert E, LaDu TJ, Cohen J (1986) Anorexia nervosa. Treatment efficacy of cyproheptadine and amitriptyline. *Arch Gen Psychiatry* **43**: 177–81

Hamilton K, Waller G (1993) Media influences on body size estimation in anorexia and bulimia. An experimental study. *Br J Psychiatry* **162**: 837–40

Hebebrand J, Himmelmann GW, Herzog W *et al* (1997) Prediction of low body weight at long-term follow-up in acute anorexia nervosa by low body weight at referral. *Am J Psychiatry* **154**: 566–9

Heron GB, Johnston DA (1976) Hypothalamic tumor presenting as anorexia nervosa. *Am J Psychiatry* **133**: 580–2

Heron JM, Leheup therefore (1984) Happy families? *Br J Psychiatry* **145**: 136–8

Herzog W, Deter HC, Fiehn W, Petzold E (1997) Medical findings and predictors of long-term physical outcome in anorexia nervosa: a prospective, 12-year follow-up study. *Psychol Med* **27**: 269–79

Hindler CG, Norris DL (1986) A case of anorexia nervosa with Klinefelter's syndrome. *Br J Psychiatry* **149**: 659–60

Hoek HW, Bartelds AI, Bosveld JJ *et al* (1995) Impact of urbanization on detection rates of eating disorders. *Am J Psychiatry* **152**: 1272–78

Horne RL, Van Vactor JC, Emerson S (1991) Disturbed body image in patients with eating disorders. *Am J Psychiatry* **148**: 211–15

Kingston K, Szmukler G, Andrewes D, Tress B, Desmond P (1996) Neuropsychological and structural brain changes in anorexia nervosa before and after refeeding. *Psychol Med* **26**: 15–28

Lilenfeld LR, Kaye WH, Greeno CG *et al* (1998) A controlled family study of anorexia nervosa and bulimia nervosa: psychiatric disorders in first-degree relatives and effects of proband comorbidity. *Arch Gen Psychiatry* **55**: 603–10

McCluskey SE, Lacey JH (1992) Anorexia nervosa in a patient with XY gonadal dysgenesis. *Br J Psychiatry* **160**: 114–6

Mehler PS (1996) Bone density in amenorrheic athletes and in anorexia nervosa. *J Am Med Ass* **276**: 1384

Oldham JM, Skodol AE, Kellman HD *et al* (1995) Comorbidity of axis I and axis II disorders. *Am J Psychiatry* **152**: 571–8

Palazidou E, Robinson P, Lishman WA (1990) Neuroradiological and neuropsychological assessment in anorexia nervosa. *Psychol Med* **20**: 521–7

Park RJ, Lawrie SM, Freeman CP (1995) Post-viral onset of anorexia nervosa. *Br J Psychiatry* **166**: 386–9

Patton GC, Wood K, Johnson-Sabine E (1986) Physical illness. A risk factor in anorexia nervosa. *Br J Psychiatry* **149**: 756–9

Patton GC, Johnson-Sabine E, Wood K, Mann AH, Wakeling A (1990) Abnormal eating attitudes in London schoolgirls — a prospective epidemiological study: outcome at twelve-month follow-up. *Psychol Med* **20**: 383–94

Powers PS (1982) Heart failure during treatment of anorexia nervosa. *Am J Psychiatry* **139**: 1167–70

Ratcliffe PJ, Bevan JS (1985) Severe hypoglycaemia and sudden death in anorexia nervosa. *Psychol Med* **15**: 679–81

Rosenvinge JH, Mouland SO (1990) Outcome and prognosis of anorexia nervosa. A retrospective study of 41 subjects. *Br J Psychiatry* **156**: 92–7

Russell GFM, Szmukler GI, Dare C, Eisler I (1987) An evaluation of family therapy in anorexia nervosa and bulimia nervosa. *Arch Gen Psychiatry* **44**: 1047–56

Rutherford J, McGuffin P, Katz RJ, Murray RM (1993) Genetic influences on eating attitudes in a normal female twin population. *Psychol Med* **23**: 425–36

Salisbury JJ, Mitchell JE (1991) Bone mineral density and anorexia nervosa in women. *Am J Psychiatry* **148**: 768–74

Schmidt U, Evans K, Tiller J, Treasure J (1995) Puberty, sexual milestones and abuse: how are they related in eating disorder patients? *Psychol Med* **25**: 413–7

Schmidt U, Tiller J, Blanchard M, Andrews B, Treasure J (1997) Is there a specific trauma precipitating anorexia nervosa? *Psychol Med* **27**: 523–30

Sharp CW, Freeman CP (1993) The medical complications of anorexia nervosa. *Br J Psychiatry* **162**: 452–62

Slade PD (1977) Awareness of body dimensions during pregnancy: an analogue study. *Psychol Med* **7**: 245–52

Sours JA (1983) Case reports of anorexia nervosa and caffeinism. *Am J Psychiatry* **140**: 235–6

Srinivasagam NM, Kaye WH, Plotnicov KH, Greeno C, Weltzin TE, Rao R (1995) Persistent perfectionism, symmetry, and exactness after long-term recovery from anorexia nervosa. *Am J Psychiatry* **152**: 1630–4

Steel JM, Young RJ, Lloyd GG, Macintyre CC (1989) Abnormal eating attitudes in young insulin-dependent diabetics. *Br J Psychiatry* **155**: 515–21

Strober M, Goldenberg I, Green J, Saxon J (1979) Body image disturbance in anorexia nervosa during the acute and recuperative phase. *Psychol Med* **9**: 695–701

Sullivan PF, Bulik CM, Fear JL, Pickering A (1998) Outcome of anorexia nervosa: a case-control study. *Am J Psychiatry* **155**: 939–46

Swayze VW 2nd, Andersen A, Arndt S *et al* (1996) Reversibility of brain tissue loss in anorexia nervosa assessed with a computerized Talairach 3-D proportional grid. *Psychol Med* **26**: 381–90

Szmukler GI, Eisler I, Russell GF, Dare C (1985) Anorexia nervosa, parental 'expressed emotion' and dropping out of treatment. *Br J Psychiatry* **147**: 265–71

Thiel A, Broocks A, Ohlmeier M, Jacoby GE, Schussler G (1995) Obsessive-compulsive disorder among patients with anorexia nervosa and bulimia nervosa. *Am J Psychiatry* **152**: 72–5

Thomas CS, Harris B (1982) Anorexia nervosa following termination of pregnancy. *Br J Psychiatry* **141**: 428

Touyz SW, O'Sullivan BT, Gertler R, Beumont PJ (1988) Anorexia nervosa in a woman totally blind since birth. *Br J Psychiatry* **153**: 248–50

Touyz SW, Lennerts W, Freeman RJ, Beumont PJ (1990) To weigh or not to weigh? Frequency of weighing and rate of weight gain in patients with anorexia nervosa. *Br J Psychiatry* **157**: 752–4

Troop NA, Treasure JL (1997) Setting the scene for eating disorders, II. Childhood helplessness and mastery. *Psychol Med* **27**: 531–8

Vandereycken W (1984) Neuroleptics in the short-term treatment of anorexia nervosa. A double-blind placebo-controlled study with sulpiride. *Br J Psychiatry* **144**: 288–92

van der Ham T, Meulman JJ, van Strien DC, van Engeland H (1997) Empirically based subgrouping of eating disorders in adolescents: a longitudinal perspective. *Br J Psychiatry* **170**: 363–8

Vize CM, Cooper PJ (1995) Sexual abuse in patients with eating disorder, patients with depression, and normal controls. A comparative study. *Br J Psychiatry* **167**: 80–5

Wamboldt FS, Kaslow NJ, Swift WJ, Ritholz M)1987) Short-term course of depressive symptoms in patients with eating disorders. *Am J Psychiatry* **144**: 362–4

Warren SE, Steinberg SM (1979) Acid-base and electrolyte disturbances in anorexia nervosa. *Am J Psychiatry* **136**(4A): 415–8

Weller RA, Weller EB (1982) Anorexia nervosa in a patient with an infiltrating tumor of the hypothalamus. *Am J Psychiatry* **139**: 824–5

Weltzin TE, Fernstrom MH, Hansen D, McConaha C, Kaye WH (1991) Abnormal caloric requirements for weight maintenance in patients with anorexia and bulimia nervosa. *Am J Psychiatry* **148**: 1675–82

White JH, Kelly P, Dorman K (1977) Clinical picture of atypical anorexia nervosa associated with hypothalamic tumor. *Am J Psychiatry* **134**: 323–5

Wichstrom L (1995) Social, psychological and physical correlates of eating problems. A study of the general adolescent population in Norway. *Psychol Med* **25**: 567–79

Windauer U, Lennerts W, Talbot P, Touyz SW, Beumont PJ (1993) How well are 'cured' anorexia nervosa patients? An investigation of 16 weight-recovered anorexic patients. *Br J Psychiatry* **163**: 195–200

Yager J, Hatton CA, Ma L (1986) Anorexia nervosa in a woman totally blind since the age of two. *Br J Psychiatry* **149**: 506–9

Further reading

American Psychiatric Association (1993) Practice guideline for eating disorders. *Am J Psychiatry* **150**: 212–8

Ploog DW, Pirke KM (1987) Psychobiology of anorexia nervosa. *Psychol Med* **17**: 843–59

3

Anxiety disorders

History of presenting complaint

1. History of previous episodes of anxiety or treatment for anxiety

2. Life event that may have precipitated this episode

3. Type of anxiety syndrome

Generalised anxiety disorder (ICD-10)

- ◆ 'Free-floating' anxiety
- ◆ Apprehension
    - ❑ worries about future misfortunes
    - ❑ feeling 'on edge'
- ◆ Motor tension
    - ❑ restless fidgeting
    - ❑ tension headaches
    - ❑ inability to relax
- ◆ Autonomic over activity
    - ❑ lightheadedness
    - ❑ sweating
    - ❑ tachycardia/tachypnoea
    - ❑ epigastric discomfort
    - ❑ dizziness
    - ❑ dry mouth

Panic attacks/disorder (ICD-10)

Panic attack

- ◆ Episodes of sudden onset of
    - ❑ intense anxiety
    - ❑ palpitations
    - ❑ chest pain, shortness of breath
    - ❑ choking sensation
    - ❑ dizziness
    - ❑ trembling/shaking

  ❏ feelings of unreality
    derealisation / depersonalisation
- Secondary fear that having a heart attack, of dying, losing control or going mad
- Sense of imminent danger or impending doom, hurried exit from the site where the person is and avoidance of return there.

Agoraphobia
- Fear of crowded places and escape from them
- Avoidance of the places.

Phobia

Simple phobia
- Intense fear of an object or a situation that would not in itself be expected to cause fear
- Recognition that the fear is irrational
- Anticipatory avoidance.

Most frequent objects of a phobia are animals, heights, thunder, darkness, flying, closed spaces, urinating or defaecating in public places, eating certain foods, dentistry, the sight of blood or injury, the fear of exposure to certain illnesses (ICD-10)

Social phobia (ICD-10)
- Fear of scrutiny by others in small groups
- Avoidance of social situations leading to social isolation
- Blushing, tremor, nausea, urgency of micturition

4. Associated psychiatric disorder

- Depressive illness
- Obsessive compulsive disorder
- Alcohol/substance abuse
- Dementia
- Schizophrenia

5. Complications resulting from the symptoms

Social

- Loss of days at school
- Loss of days at work; failure to obtain promotion; inability to carry out a job when travel is required; loss of job
- Loss of important relationships
- Loss of ability to go out of the house or travel on public transport

Psychological

- Secondary demoralisation
- Secondary psychiatric disorder

6. Precipitant/reason for presentation

Family history

- Family history of anxiety disorder
- Conflict between parents
- Conflict of patient with parents
- Physical abuse
- Sexual abuse.

Personal history

- Shyness in childhood
- Well-behaved child
    - less disciplinary difficulty
    - less theft
    - less running away or fights
- Under performance at school
- Higher education
- Evidence of social impairment
    - giving up job (especially if due to illness)
    - under performance in career
    - (others — see above)

Past medical history

- Asthma
- Hypertension
- Hyperthyroidism
- Hyperparathyroidism
- Phaeochromocytoma
- Vestibular dysfunction
- Seizure disorders
- Cardiac conditions
    - arrhythmias
    - supraventricular tachycardia
    - mitral valve prolapse
- Temporal lobe epilepsy

- Hypoglycaemia
  - insulinoma
  - hypoglycaemia in insulin-dependent diabetes.

Past psychiatric history

- Associated psychiatric illnesses (see above)
- Substance abuse
  - direct toxic effect of CNS stimulants
    cocaine; amphetamine; cannabis; caffeine
  - withdrawal syndrome from CNS depressants
    alcohol; barbiturates; benzodiazepines; opiates.

Drug history

- Drugs that might give rise to symptoms of anxiety
  - thyroid replacement therapy
  - insulin
- History of drugs used to treat anxiety
  - benzodiazepines
  - propranolol.

Pre-morbid personality

- Socially anxious
- Hypersensitivity to criticism, negative evaluation and rejection
- Few friends
- Dependent
- Immature.

Social circumstances

- Living alone; may still be with parents, although an adult may be married.

Psychosexual history

- May be married, but spouse/partner may have given up job to care.

Mental state examination

Appearance

- Strained face, furrowed brow
- Tense, restless, fine tremor
- Pale skin
- Sweaty hands

Behaviour

- Anxious posture
- Inability to keep still
- Fidgeting
- Conveys sense of being frightened or 'impending doom'
- May be 'clingy' and grasp the interviewer as though 'begging' for help — mildly histrionic
- May come across as demanding or manipulative.

Mood

- Anxious; depressed feelings with biological symptoms when depression supervenes.

Affect

- Anxious appearance.

Speech

- Normal grammar, speed, volume. May have an anxious tremor to it. The patient may complain of some difficulty with articulation due to a dry mouth (secondary to hyper-ventilation).

Thoughts

- Only suicidal if finding situation hard to cope with, or if supervening depression
- Low self-esteem, with difficulty in being assertive
- Some feelings of guilt.

Experiences

- Hallucinations and delusions are absent.

Cognition

- Intact (in the absence of underlying dementia).

Insight

- ◆ Intact. The patient is aware that the fears are irrational, but is unable to do anything about it.

Investigations

- ◆ Informant history and case notes
    - ❑ past episodes
    - ❑ psychosocial environment (eg. family situation)
- ◆ urine, blood and physiological tests to exclude organic pathology
    - ❑ urine
      dipstick for glucose and ketones; urine drug screen
    - ❑ blood
      thyroid function tests
    - ❑ physiological
      ECG; peak flow meter; EEG

Management

Pharmacological

- ◆ Benzodiazepines (short-term only)
- ◆ β-adrenoceptor antagonists
    - ❑ propranolol
- ◆ Antidepressant drugs
    - ❑ tricyclic antidepressants
    - ❑ monoamine oxidase inhibitors
    - ❑ SSRIs
- ◆ Low dose neuroleptic medication

Psychological

- ◆ Simple explanation
- ◆ Support
- ◆ Self-help books
- ◆ Counselling
- ◆ Relaxation training
- ◆ Paper bag for hyperventilation
- ◆ Assertiveness training
- ◆ Social skill training

- Systematic desensitisation
- Cognitive-behavioural therapy
- Psychotherapy.

Social

- Outpatient treatment
  - surgery
  - CPN visits
- Day hospital treatment

✱ ✱ ✱ ✱ ✱

Before an examination; before you are about to go out on a date with someone you really fancy; before your wedding (or just as you are about to go on bended knee to propose...); before you are about to go into the room for the interview for the job you really want. The feelings well-known: butterflies in the pit of your stomach, which is churning; feeling hot, bothered and sweaty; repeatedly wanting to go to the loo and feeling anxious. Then, when it is over, these anxious feelings have vanished (and if successful given way to elation).

Anxiety is normal not only in humans, but also in other species. It is how the mind knows that there is a problem (or a threat) to be dealt with. It may be a danger (such as a predator) or a challenge. It tells the animal that there is an impending problem and the physical concomitants prepare the body for additional physical effort (eg. to fight or to run hard).

However, as with any other mechanism in the body (physical or mental), it can function inappropriately and this is noted in a medical disorder. There can be too much or too little anxiety; it can be inappropriate (eg. being anxious about the presence of a spider when the spider does not represent a threat); or in can last longer than is appropriate. All these lead to patients visiting their doctor with their complaints. When anxiety, and the patient's response to it, interferes with the normal activities of daily life, then anxiety can be regarded as abnormal and deserves medical consideration.

Anxiety can cause distress for the sufferer and those listening to the sufferer's complaint. It can be aggravated by the patient's genuine distress, which the listener may dismiss as 'neurotic' (in the lay sense). Frequently, this arises when the patient and the listener (friend, doctor or other professional) views what is happening in different ways. For example, the patient may focus on the unpleasant experience of the anxiety, whereas the listener may recognise that the solution is straightforward and be less than sympathetic.

As an unpleasant emotion, people who experience anxiety want to be free of it. In appropriate anxiety in an acute situation, such as that mentioned above, the sensible approach is to deal with the matter, ie. by taking the driving test, speaking in public, carrying out the challenging task, or whatever stress is occurring, and then allowing the anxiety to subside. The anxiety is seen as normal, as is the action taken to resolve it. However, some people focus not on the overall situation, but on the anxiety and they try to avoid the unpleasant experience of anxiety itself. To relieve the anxiety, a person may take an alcoholic drink, refuse to carry on with the planned activity (such as give a public speech), leave the room, fail to turn up at the venue, or throw the bill in the bin. The feeling of anxiety is swiftly and promptly removed, but the threat or challenge is not faced, and the situation that gave rise to the anxiety is likely to recur. A person listening to the complainant may become exasperated as the solution appears simple. Although the solution may be obvious to others, it is not so for the person concerned , otherwise the situation would have been resolved. Helping a person to avoid anxiety-producing situations involves helping him/her to realise what is happening, and to learn how to deal with the anxiety-producing situation more appropriately. This process is not eased by patronising or demeaning the anxious person.

There are several forms of chronic anxiety:

- **people who are anxious all the time**, without any apparent cause for the anxiety. The patient is described as having **free-floating anxiety**. There is no obvious precipitant. People who feel anxious in this way are described as suffering from a generalised anxiety disorder.

- **people who are anxious about one particular thing**, such as a spider, blood, vomiting, becoming ill, or thunderstorms. The anxiety may be quite out of proportion to the threat that the object presents to the person. This is referred to as a phobia. In theory, a person may develop a phobia about anything, but items mentioned above and in the clinical case part of this section are particularly common. If they suspect they may encounter a situation that is likely to provoke this anxiety, they may become anxious (**anticipatory anxiety**) and they go out of their way to avoid the situation, sometimes going to great lengths (**avoidance behaviour**)

- **those experiencing episodes of sudden panic onset**, followed by intense fear and awareness of physical changes, such as increased heart rate, dry mouth, dizziness, sweating, numbness and tingling. The episode may last from a few minutes to a few hours and is referred to as a **panic attack**. Those who experiences a number of panic attacks are said to suffer from **panic disorder**. A common occurrence is in people who are prone to panic attacks when in crowded or public places. They may bolt from a supermarket in a dramatic manner and subsequently cease from going shopping. In extreme cases, they refuse to leave the house in case they suffer from a repeat attack. This is referred to as **agoraphobia**. If patients refuse to leave the house because of the risk of experiencing a panic attack, this could mean that someone else must do the tasks or chores that are otherwise the responsibility of the patient. For example, a female patient suffering from agoraphobia may refuse to go out to do the shopping and her husband may be forced to take over the responsibility for doing the weekly shop. In this way, through her psychological disability, she persuades her husband to do the task that she does not want to do. A benefit obtained by a person **as a result** of a psychological disorder is referred to as a **secondary gain** and those who obtain such benefits are frequently regarded contemptuously by others. They may be described as 'manipulative, 'acting' or 'pulling a fast one', etc.

From these descriptions, it is not surprising that patients presenting with anxiety disorders are unpopular with doctors and other health and social professionals. It is not the role of these professionals to criticise patients, but rather to assess the condition and offer whatever medical and/or social help available. The professional should learn how to handle the patient's behaviour, Whether it is manipulative, demanding, immature or dependent, excessive use of scarce resources, ie. the doctor's time, or potential or actual violent behaviour, the professional must control the aggressive and distasteful emotions generated in him/her self by such conduct. The professional will need support from his or her colleagues and from the management of the organisation by whom he/she is employed. The temptation to dismiss the patient without giving available treatment, or giving technically poor treatment should be firmly resisted.

Initially, the patient should be assessed to see whether he/she is showing evidence of avoiding normal anxiety or is suffering from an anxiety disorder, ie. generalised anxiety disorder, phobia or panic disorder. If the anxiety is thought to be pathological, the doctor should test for those medical disorders that either mimic anxiety disorders or have anxiety as a common symptom, for example, thyrotoxicosis.

Having diagnosed the patient as not suffering from an underlying medical condition, there are a range of treatment options that can be grouped together as drug treatments and psychological treatments. A good basic review of these options is given by Lader (1994). Both drug and psychological treatments have a role to play. The professional should know which treatment to select for the patient, during the course of a condition that may last for weeks, months or even years.

As anxiety disorders have the potential for cure or substantial remission, this should be the overall aim of management by the professional. To achieve this often requires psychological change, which may take some time. Psychological treatment is likely to be more effective. Meanwhile, the patient is experiencing distress, emotional discomfort and many social problems. The continuing anxiety and associated psychological problem, such as depression, alcohol abuse or repeated suicide attempts, could be reduced in the short-term while the process of psychological treatment is tried. Social problems arising out of damage to relationships with partner and family, an inability to do housework or take up paid employment (with a consequential risk of loss of accommodation, poor nutrition, etc) need aid. The skill of the professional is to judge whether short- or long-term intervention is necessary. This requires the ability to identify when short-term interventions will impede the development of long-term change and recovery, and also the ability to resist demands for short-term intervention, seen by the patient as a 'solution' when it is only a stop-gap remedy.

Keeping these principles in mind, a rational approach can be taken to select the appropriate intervention. When the patient first presents to a doctor or at times of acute exacerbation of anxiety it may be appropriate to use a medication, such as a benzodiazepine (eg. valium) to alleviate the distress short-term. If the distress lasts longer than a few weeks, then a change to an antidepressant medication may be more appropriate, partly because of the risk of benzodiazepine dependence. Dependence on benzodiazepines can itself cause serious problems (Higgitt *et al*, 1985), but this group of drugs is much safer than the barbiturates that were prescribed originally, and a sense of perspective is needed (Kräupl Taylor, 1989). When the patient's ability to care for him/herself is impaired, or when a high-level of supervision is required, psychiatric hospital in patient admission may be appropriate, but this should only be for a few days. In the absence of an acute crisis, intensive support can be provided by a day hospital.

These measures only provide brief symptomatic relief. They help patients who have difficulty accepting the psychological components to their anxiety and who are reluctant to consider psychological treatment.

Not all patients suffer from symptoms severe enough to require hospital admission or drug therapy. For many, simple psychological techniques, such as counselling, relaxation training or systematic desensitisation (assisting a patient with a phobia to manage the phobic stimulus) are effective. For those with more severe symptoms, a deeper understanding of the psychological basis of their symptoms may be gained by using techniques, such as individual psychotherapy. It may take months or years for a person who has severe symptoms to learn to recognise them, and other supportive measures should be used during this time.

Further reading

den Boer JA (1997) Social phobia: epidemiology, recognition and treatment. *Br Med J* **315**: 796–800

Hale AS (1997) Anxiety. *Br Med J* **314**: 1886–9

Higgitt AC, Lader MH, Fonagy P (1985) Clinical management of benzodiazepine dependence. *Br Med J* **291**: 688–90

Kräupl Taylor F (1989) The damnation of benzodiazepines. *Br J Psychiatry* **154**: 697–704

Lader M (1994) Treatment of anxiety. *Br Med J* **309**: 321–4

History of presenting complaint

Although it appears that many precursors to adult-onset anxiety disorders are present in the family of origin and in childhood (see below), nevertheless, the patient will not develop a clinically manifest disorder until adulthood. Such disorders usually begin between the ages of 18 and 35 years. There is evidence that stressful life events, such as financial difficulties or arguments, can precipitate the onset of the disorder (Angst and Vollrath, 1991).

The three different types of anxiety disorder referred to in this chapter should be sought independently, but in clinical practice there is often comorbidity between them; for example, one study found that 87% of a sample of 164 patients with DSM-III-R generalised anxiety disorder had another anxiety disorder, most frequently panic disorder with agoraphobia or social phobia (Yonkers *et al*, 1996). There is evidence that supports the current classification of agoraphobia as a variant of panic disorder, but suggests that it is distinct from other affective disorders (Noyes *et al*, 1986).

Anxiety disorders often have a poor prognosis, with many developing a mixed anxiety-depression picture and/or additional substance abuse over a period of years (Angst and Vollrath, 1991). Thus, although anxiety may be secondary to another major psychiatric illness, such as schizophrenia or dementia, or even a direct effect of chronic alcohol consumption (ie. alcoholism causes anxiety disorder, especially panic disorder and generalised anxiety disorder, and is not just a form of self-medication of anxiety [Mullan *et al*, 1986; Kushner *et al*, 1990]), depression and substance abuse seem to be frequent secondary complications of anxiety disorders.

Family history

Family studies show a that first degree relatives have a prevalence of anxiety neurosis six to eight times that of controls. The concordance rate for anxiety neurosis for monozygotic twins is 56% compared with 40% for dizygotic twins. The lifetime morbidity risk for definite panic disorder in first degree relatives of probands is 17% compared with 2% in controls. In phobic disorders, one study showed 7/8 monozygotic and 5/13 dizygotic twins concordant (Marks, 1986).

There have been various theories that people with anxiety disorders show a greater autonomic responsiveness than those without, and such a response may be the basis of an inherited component. For example, it has recently been shown that those patients who have a hypersensitivity to carbon dioxide challenge, responding with a panic attack, are more likely to have a family history of panic disorder than those who do not (Perna *et al*, 1996).

There is evidence that certain psychosocial features of the family of origin increase the risk of anxiety disorders: conflict between parents, conflict with parents, sexual trauma and lack of attention all occur more frequently in the families of patients than controls (Angst and Vollrath, 1991); physical abuse in children of both sexes and sexual abuse in women (Stein *et al*, 1996, where the anxiety sample contained patients with OCD as well as panic disorder and social phobia).

It has been observed in a small study that patients with generalised anxiety disorder have an increased incidence of loss of a parent before the age of 16 years, compared to patients with panic disorder and agoraphobia (Torgersen, 1986).

The relationship between anxiety disorders and parental or familial alcohol abuse is uncertain. Several studies have suggested an increase of alcohol disorders in relatives of people with agoraphobia (eg. Noyes *et al*, 1986), and that the adult children of alcoholics have a higher incidence of a number of psychiatric disorders including: dysthymia; anxiety disorders (generalised anxiety disorder, simple phobia, panic disorder and agoraphobia); antisocial symptoms and alcohol and drug abuse in males (Mathew *et al*, 1993). However, it seems that while anxiety disorders and depressive disorders may occur together in individuals, these disorders do not cosegregate in families, and in separating out the disorders in probands, it has been suggested that dysthymia, substance abuse and antisocial personality may show a familial connection to early-onset major depressive disorders, but not to panic disorder (Goldstein *et al*, 1994).

Personal history

In childhood, patients often have a history of being exceptionally well-behaved, and have less frequent incidences of disciplinary difficulties in school, thefts, running away or fights (Angst and Vollrath, 1991). There may have been a history of separation anxiety (Breier *et al*, 1986). Subjects with anxiety are over represented among persons with higher education (Angst and Vollrath, 1991).

Past medical history

This section is relevant for three reasons. Several medical conditions may present with anxiety as a component, and these must be detected and treated. This may be followed by a remission in the anxiety disorder. Secondly, certain physical illnesses have a presentation similar to anxiety disorders, and these must be considered as part of the differential diagnosis. Thirdly, anxiety disorders are associated with and at times aetiological in the development of physical illness.

- **mitral valve prolapse** is not infrequently associated with anxiety disorders, although the causal relationship between these two conditions has not been clarified (Dager *et al*, 1988)
- **anxiety disorders**, mainly agoraphobia, but also generalised anxiety disorder can be precipitated by stroke. For such patients who have co-morbid depression, mortality is higher (Burvill *et al*, 1995)
- anxiety can be a symptom of hyperthyroidism (Heinik, 1986), phaeochromocytoma (Mackenzie and Popkin, 1983), insulinoma, pituitary microadenoma (Wilcox, 1991) and acute porphyria (Elder *et al*, 1997).

There is also an increased incidence of phobias in female patients with Type I diabetes mellitus compared to the general population (Popkin *et al*, 1988). Community instruments of anxiety and depression are predictive of later hypertension diagnosis and pharmacological treatment (Jonas *et al*, 1997). There is also evidences of a relation between phobic anxiety and fatal ischaemic heart disease (Haines *et al*, 1987). There is an association between asthma and panic disorder that is greater than might be expected (Shavitt *et al*, 1992), and with other anxiety disorders. Among patients with hypertension or diabetes mellitus, those who have comorbid anxiety disorders are more debilitated than patients who do not (Sherbourne *et al*, 1996).

There is evidence that panic disorder may lead to increased mortality from heart disease (Nutt and Lawson, 1992). There is evidence that patients with panic disorder have raised cholesterol levels (Bajwa *et al*, 1992).

Increased mortality is identified in patients with neurotic disorder (anxiety and depressive symptoms in primary care setting) from cardiovascular, respiratory and malignant diseases (Lloyd *et al*, 1996), and for patients with a psychiatric diagnosis of anxiety neurosis or depressive neurosis. As well as an increased risk of death from suicide, there was a raised risk of death from ischaemic heart disease, traumatic injury, obstructive airways disease (possibly reflecting the effects of tobacco smoking) and alcohol abuse and liver cirrhosis (Allgulander, 1994).

Past psychiatric history

Anxiety disorders often occur in conjunction with other psychiatric disorders, patients with generalised anxiety disorder frequently experiencing comorbid major depressive disorder, and patients with panic disorder frequently abusing alcohol (Massion *et al*, 1993). Some studies have found an association with obsessive-compulsive disorder (Breier *et al*,1986). Many patients with panic disorder have a history of attempted suicide, especially those with co-morbid major depression or alcohol and/or other substance abuse, both of which are commonly associated with panic disorder. Women who are single, divorced, or widowed were associated with increased risk of suicide attempt (Lepine *et al*, 1993).

The relationship with alcohol is complex. There is objective evidence of alcohol being effective as an anxiolytic in both normal subjects (Logue *et al*, 1978) and in patients with panic disorder (Kushner *et al*, 1996). There is evidence that panic disorder and generalised anxiety disorder may follow pathological alcohol abuse; patients with agoraphobia and social phobia use alcohol as self-medication; there is no relation with simple phobia (Kushner *et al*, 1990), but several different ways in which anxiety and alcohol abuse interact have been identified (Schuckit and Hesselbrock, 1994).

Pre-morbid personality

Patients with anxiety disorders show pre-morbid personality traits of social anxiety, hypersensitivity to criticism, dependence, immaturity, hysteria and anergia (Angst and Vollrath, 1991). There is an increased risk of comorbidity of anxiety disorders with borderline, avoidant and dependent personality disorders (Oldham *et al*, 1995).

The outcome of treatment for panic disorder with benzodiazepines shows a strong and negative association with DSM-III antisocial, borderline, histrionic and narcissistic personality disorders (Reich, 1988). An association between nicotine dependence and anxiety disorders has also been identified (Breslau *et al*, 1993).

There is evidence that caffeine can cause symptoms of anxiety in patients with panic disorder, who are more sensitive than controls to the effects of caffeine (Charney *et al*, 1985); patients with panic disorder report exacerbated anxiety and panic attacks triggered by caffeine consumption (Breier *et al*, 1986).

Social circumstances

Even accounting for the contribution of family and personal factors, there was an excess of anxiety disorder and substance use among young people who have been unemployed for more than six months (Fergusson *et al*, 1997). Other psychosocial impairments found among patients with panic disorder include impaired social and marital functioning, financial dependency (Markowitz *et al*, 1989).

Management

Panic disorder and agoraphobia

In the acute treatment of panic disorder and agoraphobia, there is some evidence that diazepam has been found to be effective in a way that propranolol is not (Noyes *et al*, 1994), and which is consistent with experimental evidence that suggests propranolol does not prevent lactate-induced panic (Gorman *et al*, 1983). Exposure instruction has also been advocated for treatment of patients presenting with panic attacks to the emergency-room and found to be more effective than re-assurance (Swinson *et al*, 1992).

There is evidence to show that, for a group of patients with panic disorder, especially those without personality disorder or substance abuse supervening, the combination of behavioural counselling and treatment with antidepressant medication is efficacious. In a follow-up study of 68 patients with panic disorder, 34% were recovered and remained well and 46% were minimally impaired at five to six years (O'Rourke *et al*, 1996). Other evidence suggests that the addition of brief dynamic psychotherapy to clomipramine results in a lower relapse rate than clomipramine alone (Wiborg and Dahl, 1996). However, if patients with agoraphobia are to experience a favourable course over 2 years when treated with exposure therapy and imipramine, the response is likely to be evident in the first month (Mavissakalian and Michelson, 1986); a group of chronic agoraphobic patients were found to have responded poorly to imipramine, although they did derive some benefits from self-exposure homework or therapist-aided exposure (Marks *et al*, 1983). Alprazolam can also be helpful in reducing panic, but two and a half year follow-up of patients treated with alprazolam and a behavioural group treatment programme found that, although frequency of panic attack remained as low as on discharge from the programme, episodes of major depression were common (Nagy *et al*, 1989). Other studies have found a greater effect size acutely for exposure than for alprazolam and, in the longer term, gains from exposure therapy persisting for six months after stopping treatment, but no gain once alprazolam was stopped (Marks *et al*, 1993).

Other psychotherapeutic treatments that have been considered for use in patients with panic disorder include focused cognitive therapy (Beck *et al*, 1992) and psychodynamic psychotherapy (Milrod *et al*, 1996). There is some suggestion that the use of meditation might be helpful in the management of patients with anxiety disorders (Kabat-Zinn *et al*, 1992).

Generalised anxiety disorder

Anxiolytic drugs have been used in generalised anxiety disorder. In the short-term (the first two weeks), benzodiazepines are helpful, but over the course of ten weeks, dothiepin, cognitive behavioural therapy and self-help techniques give better results than placebo, but diazepam results are worse (Tyrer *et al*, 1988).

There is evidence that psychological therapies are helpful. Anxiety management (including a booklet explaining about the origins of anxiety symptoms, relaxation exercises, distraction techniques, control of upsetting thoughts and techniques to raise self-confidence) has been shown to be effective (Butler *et al*, 1987). In primary care and non-psychiatric populations, psychological therapies, such as cognitive therapy, have been shown to be effective in maintaining gains over three months (Durham and Allan, 1993); in secondary care, anxiety management (even provided by trainee psychiatrists) and cognitive therapy has been shown to provide a more sustained effect over six months than brief dynamic psychotherapy. Treatment of eight to ten sessions is as effective as 16–20 sessions (Durham *et al*, 1994).

Phobia

There is evidence of the efficacy of exposure treatments, both as a self-help technique and supported by a therapist (Ghosh *et al*, 1988).

References

Allgulander C (1994) Suicide and mortality patterns in anxiety neurosis and depressive neurosis. *Arch Gen Psychiatry* **51**: 708–12

Angst J, Vollrath M (1991) The natural history of anxiety disorders. *Acta Psych Scand* **84**: 446–52

Bajwa WK, Asnis GM, Sanderson WC, Irfan A, van Praag HM (1992) High cholesterol levels in patients with panic disorder. *Am J Psychiatry* **149**: 376–8

Beck AT, Sokol L, Clark DA, Berchick R, Wright F (1992) A crossover study of focused cognitive therapy for panic disorder. *Am J Psychiatry* **149**: 778–3

Breier A, Charney DS, Heninger GR (1986) Agoraphobia with panic attacks. Development, diagnostic stability, and course of illness. *Arch Gen Psychiatry* **43**: 1029–36

Breslau N, Kilbey MM, Andreski P (1993) Vulnerability to psychopathology in nicotine-dependent smokers: an epidemiologic study of young adults. *Am J Psychiatry* **150**: 941–6

Burvill PW, Johnson GA, Jamrozik KD, Anderson CS, Stewart-Wynne EG, Chakera TMH (1995) Anxiety disorders after stroke: results from the Perth Community stroke study. *Br J Psychiatry* **166**: 328

Butler G, Cullington A, Hibbert G, Klimes I, Gelder M.(1987) Anxiety management for persistent generalised anxiety. *Br J Psychiatry* **151**: 535–42

Charney DS, Heninger GR, Jatlow PI (1985) Increased anxiogenic effects of caffeine in panic disorders. *Arch Gen Psychiatry* **42**: 233–43

Dager SR, Saal AK, Comess KA, Dunner DL (1988) Mitral valve prolapse and the anxiety disorders. *Hos Comm Psychiatry* **39**: 517–27

Durham RC, Allan T (1993) Psychological treatment of generalised anxiety disorder. A review of the clinical significance of results in outcome studies since 1980. *Br J Psychiatry* **163**: 19–26

Durham RC, Murphy T, Allan T, Richard K, Treliving LR, Fenton GW (1994) Cognitive therapy, analytic psychotherapy and anxiety management training for generalised anxiety disorder. *Br J Psychiatry* **165**: 315–23

Elder GH, Hift RJ, Meissner PN (1997) The acute porphyrias. *Lancet* **349**: 1613–7

Fergusson DM, Horwood LJ, Lynskey MT (1997) The effects of unemployment on psychiatric illness during young adulthood. *Psychol Med* **27**: 371–81

Ghosh A, Marks IM, Carr AC (1988) Therapist contact and outcome of self-exposure treatment for phobias: a controlled study. *Br J Psychiatry* **152**: 234–8

Goldstein RB, Weissman MM, Adams PB *et al* (1994) Psychiatric disorders in relatives of probands with panic disorder and/or major depression. *Arch Gen Psychiatry* **51**: 383–94

Gorman JM, Levy GF, Liebowitz MR *et al* (1983) Effect of acute beta-adrenergic blockade on lactate-induced panic. *Arch Gen Psychiatry* **40**: 1079–82

Haines AP, Imeson JD, Meade TW (1987) Phobic anxiety and ischaemic heart disease. *Br Med J* **295**: 297–9

Heinik J (1986) Hyperthyroidism and the organic anxiety syndrome. *Am J Psychiatry* **143**: 1497–8

Jonas BS; Franks P; Ingram DD (1997) Are symptoms of anxiety and depression risk factors for hypertension? Longitudinal evidence from the national health and nutrition examination survey epidemiologic follow-up study. *Arch Fam Med* **6**: 43–9

Kabat-Zinn J, Massion AO, Kristeller J *et al* (1992) Effectiveness of a meditation-based stress reduction program in the treatment of anxiety disorders. *Am J Psychiatry* **149**: 936–43

Kushner MG, Mackenzie TB, Fiszdon J *et al* (1996) The effects of alcohol consumption on laboratory-induced panic and state anxiety. *Arch Gen Psychiatry* **53**: 264–70

Kushner MG, Sher KJ, Beitman BD (1990) The relation between alcohol problems and the anxiety disorders. *Am J Psychiatry* **147**: 685–95

Lepine JP, Chignon JM, Teherani M (1993) Suicide attempts in patients with panic disorder. *Arch Gen Psychiatry* **50**: 144–9

Lloyd KR, Jenkins R, Mann A (1996) Long term outcome of patients with neurotic illness in general practice. *Br Med J* **313**: 26–8

Logue PE, Gentry WD, Linnoila M, Erwin CW (1978) Effect of alcohol consumption on state anxiety changes in male and female nonalcoholics. *Am J Psychiatry* **135**: 1079–81

Mackenzie TB, Popkin MK (1983) Organic anxiety syndrome. *Am J Psychiatry* **140**: 342–4

Markowitz JS, Weissman MM, Ouellette R, Lish JD, Klerman GL (1989) Quality of life in panic disorder. *Arch Gen Psychiatry* **46**: 984–92

Marks IM, Gray S, Cohen D *et al* (1983) Imipramine and brief therapists-aided exposure in agoraphobics having self-exposure homework. *Arch Gen Psychiatry* **40**: 153–62

Marks IM (1986) Genetics of fear and anxiety disorders. *Br J Psychiatry* **149**: 406–18

Marks IM, Swinson RP, Basoglu M *et al* (1993) Alprazolam and exposure alone and combined in panic disorder with agoraphobia. A controlled study in London and Toronto. *Br J Psychiatry* **162**: 776–87

Massion AO, Warshaw MG, Keller MB (1993) Quality of life and psychiatric morbidity in panic disorder and generalized anxiety disorder. *Am J Psychiatry* **150**: 600–7

Mathew RJ, Wilson WH, Blazer DG, George LK (1993) Psychiatric disorders in adult children of alcoholics: data from the Epidemiologic Catchment Area project. *Am J Psychiatry* **150**: 793–800

Mavissakalian M, Michelson L (1986) Two-year follow-up of exposure and imipramine treatment of agoraphobia. *Am J Psychiatry* **143**: 1106–12

Milrod B, Busch FN, Hollander E, Aronson A, Siever L (1996) A 23-year-old woman with panic disorder treated with psychodynamic psychotherapy. *Am J Psychiatry* **153**: 698–703

Mullan MJ, Gurling HMD, Oppenheim BE, Murray RM (1986) The relationship between alcoholism and neurosis: evidence from a twin study. *Br J Psychiatry* **148**: 435–41

Nagy LM, Krystal JH, Woods SW, Charney DS(1989) Clinical and medication outcome after short-term alprazolam and behavioral group treatment in panic disorder. 2.5 year naturalistic follow-up study. *Arch Gen Psychiatry* **46**: 993–9

Noyes R Jr, Anderson DJ, Clancy J *et al* (1984) Diazepam and propranolol in panic disorder and agoraphobia. *Arch Gen Psychiatry* **41**: 287–92

Noyes R Jr, Crowe RR, Harris EL, Hamra BJ, McChesney CM, Chaudhry DR (1986) Relationship between panic disorder and agoraphobia. A family study. *Arch Gen Psychiatry* **43**: 227–32

Nutt D, Lawson C (1992) Panic attacks. A neurochemical overview of models and mechanisms. *Br J Psychiatry* **160**: 165–78

Oldham JM, Skodol AE, Kellman HD *et al* (1995) Comorbidity of axis I and axis II disorders. *Am J Psychiatry* **152**: 571–8

O'Rourke D, Fahy TJ, Brophy J, Prescott P (1996) The Galway Study of Panic Disorder III: Outcome at 5 to 6 years. *Br J Psychiatry* **168**: 462–9

Perna G, Bertani A, Caldirola D, Bellodi L (1996) Family history of panic disorder and hypersensitivity to CO_2 in patients with panic disorder. *Am J Psychiatry* **153**: 1060–4

Popkin MK, Callies AL, Lentz RD, Colon EA, Sutherland DE (1988)Prevalence of major depression, simple phobia, and other psychiatric disorders in patients with long-standing type I diabetes mellitus. *Arch Gen Psychiatry* **45**: 64–8

Reich JH (1988) DSM-III personality disorders and the outcome of treated panic disorder. *Am J Psychiatry* **145**: 1149–52

Schuckit MA, Hesselbrock V (1994) Alcohol dependence and anxiety disorders: what is the relationship? *Am J Psychiatry* **151**: 1723–34

Shavitt RG, Gentil V, Mandetta R (1992) The association of panic/agoraphobia and asthma: Contributing factors and clinical implications. *Gen Hos Psychiatry* **14**: 420–3

Sherbourne CD; Wells KB; Meredith LS; Jackson CA; Camp P (1996) Comorbid anxiety disorder and the functioning and well-being of chronically ill patients of general medical providers. *Arch Gen Psychiatry* **53**: 889–95

Stein MB, Walker JR, Anderson G *et al* (1996) Childhood physical and sexual abuse in patients with anxiety disorders and in a community sample. *Am J Psychiatry* **153**: 275–7

Swinson RP, Soulios C, Cox BJ, Kuch K (1992) Brief treatment of emergency room patients with panic attacks. *Am J Psychiatry* **149**: 944–6

Torgersen S (1986) Childhood and family characteristics in panic and generalized anxiety disorders. *Am J Psychiatry* **143**: 630 2

Tyrer P, Sievewright N, Murphy S *et al* (1988) The Nottingham Study of neurotic disorder: comparison of drug and psychological treatment. *Lancet* **ii**: 235–40

Wiborg IM, Dahl AA (1996) Does brief dynamic psychotherapy reduce the relapse rate of panic disorder? *Arch Gen Psychiatry* **53**: 689–94

Wilcox JA (1991) Pituitary microadenoma presenting as panic attacks. *Br J Psychiatry* **158**: 426

Yonkers KA, Warshaw MG, Massion AO, Keller MB (1996) Phenomenology and course of generalised anxiety disorder. *Br J Psychiatry* **168**:308–1

4

Dementia

History

1. Symptoms

Cognitive impairment/dementing process

- ◆ Memory defect (and extent of loss)
  - ❑ forgets that he/she has just eaten
  - ❑ puts things away and forgets where he/she put them (in some cases leading to paranoid ideas about theft)
  - ❑ leaves the gas on
  - ❑ forgets where he/she left the car
  - ❑ forgets recent events
  - ❑ forgets long-term events
  - ❑ cannot recognise acquaintances
  - ❑ cannot recognise spouse/close relative
  - ❑ talking about parents as though alive, or children as though still not adults when they are
  - ❑ repeatedly asking the same question
  - ❑ failure to recognise his/her own image in the mirror
- ◆ Dyspraxias
  - ❑ cannot find way round house/wanders
  - ❑ incontinent of urine — cannot find toilet; also frontal component of failure of control of bladder
  - ❑ cannot dress self — does not know how to put clothes on; puts clothes on inside out etc
  - ❑ cannot remember how to use a knife and fork
  - ❑ cannot cook or make a cup of tea
  - ❑ cannot wash self
  - ❑ unable to handle money or receive change
- ◆ Failure of self-care
  - ❑ neglects appearance, housework, buying food
- ◆ Performs actions of work
  - ❑ for example, a carpenter behaves as though carving wood, putting door on hinges

- Personality change
  - ❏ fatuous; aggressive; disinhibited
  - ❏ emphasis of traits of pre-morbid personality ('hardening of the personality')
  - ❏ emotional lability and irritability
  - ❏ eccentricity; repetitive and anecdotal talk
- Misperceptions
  - ❏ for example, views the bush outside the house as a person; a person on TV is perceived to be in the room
- Hypochondriacal symptoms
- Weight loss
- Loss of motivation
- Overactivity; underactivity
- Wandering, restlessness
- Epileptic fits.

Symptoms of underlying cause

2. Time course

- Sudden or gradual onset
  - ❏ precipitants (eg. following MI or CVA) or time at which a process that had already started was noticed)
  - ❏ stepwise progression
- Diurnal fluctuation
  - ❏ gradual worsening of state through the day
  - ❏ lucid periods

3. Problems that carers find intolerable

- Smearing faeces
- Incontinence
- Unpredictable aggression.

Family history

- Family history of Alzheimer's disease; Huntington's disease

Personal history

- Occupations associated with dementia
  - ❏ boxing

Past medical history

- ◆ Aetiology of the dementia
  - ❑ cardiovascular disease
    angina, MI, CVA; diabetes mellitus
  - ❑ Parkinson's disease
  - ❑ syphilis
  - ❑ AIDS
- ◆ Associated and aggravating conditions
  - ❑ kidney disease
  - ❑ liver disease
  - ❑ chest disease
  - ❑ head injury

Past psychiatric history

- ◆ Depression (for diagnosis of pseudodementia)

Drug history

- ◆ Any drug known to be able to cause cognitive impairment

Pre-morbid personality

- ◆ Personality disorder; characteristics that have 'hardened'
- ◆ Smoking — re: possibility of cardiovascular disease
- ◆ Alcohol — as a cause of dementia

Psychosexual history

- ◆ Frequent partners — unsafe sex (AIDS, syphilis)
- ◆ Homosexuality

Mental state

- ◆ Appearance
  - ❑ poor self-care
  - ❑ vacant look

- ◆ Behaviour
  - ❑ catastrophic reaction
- ◆ Mood
- ◆ Affect
  - ❑ apathy
  - ❑ euphoria
  - ❑ depression
- ◆ Speech
  - ❑ expressive dysphasia
  - ❑ nominal dysphasia
  - ❑ sensory dysphasia
  - ❑ mutism
  - ❑ perseveration
- ◆ Thoughts
  - ❑ paranoid ideas
- ◆ Experiences
  - ❑ auditory and visual hallucinations
  - ❑ misperceptions
    eg. doctor as insurance salesman
- ◆ Cognition
  - ❑ a formal examination such as the Folstein Mini-Mental State Examination would be very acceptable
- ◆ Memory
  - ❑ Babcock sentence
  - ❑ name and address (original)
  - ❑ name and address (patient's own)
  - ❑ current affairs
  - ❑ name of monarch
  - ❑ name of Prime Minister, President of the USA
  - ❑ date of World War II
  - ❑ colour of the British flag
- ◆ Attention
  - ❑ digit span
- ◆ Concentration
  - ❑ serial sevens
  - ❑ months of the year in reverse order
  - ❑ counting from one to ten (in reverse order)

- ◆ Orientation
  - ❒ date
  - ❒ place
  - ❒ time of year (season)
  - ❒ person
- ◆ Abstract thought; frontal lobe testing
  - ❒ explain a proverb
  - ❒ word generation (eg. number of words beginning with the letter S in 1 minute)
- ◆ Name common objects (a watch and its parts)
- ◆ Explain use of common objects (fridge,barometer, wardrobe)
- ◆ Identify a £1 coin
- ◆ Write own name
- ◆ Draw a clock face
- ◆ Copy figures in 2-D and 3-D
- ◆ Left/right discrimination
- ◆ Astereognosis.
- ◆ CAPE questions
  - ❒ patient's name; patient's address; patient's date of birth; today's date; place; name queen; name prime minister; name president of USA; name colours of British flag (6/10 = not demented).
- ◆ Insight
  - ❒ loss of insight

Physical examination

- ◆ Upgoing plantars
- ◆ Return of primitive reflexes - grasping, sucking
- ◆ Gait — marche a petit pas
- ◆ Foetal posture, with increased flexion, increased rigidity

Investigations

- ◆ Informant history
- ◆ Blood tests
  - ❒ FBC, ESR, B12, folate
  - ❒ U&Es, glucose, LFTs, calcium, phosphate
  - ❒ VDRL
- ◆ Chest X-ray
- ◆ EEG

- ◆ CT scan
- ◆ Psychometry
  - ❐ WAIS
  - ❐ CAMDEX

Management

- ◆ Medical
  - ❐ drugs
    tacrine; euroleptics for delusions; hallucinations; agitation; night sedation
  - ❐ nutrition
  - ❐ hydration
  - ❐ vitamin replacement
  - ❐ physical exercise
  - ❐ physiotherapy
    avoid contractures
  - ❐ treat aggravating physical factors vigorously
    urinary tract infection; respiratory tract infection, congestive cardiac failure; anaemia; hypertension
  - ❐ admission to psychogeriatric ward, relief admission, day hospital
    occupational therapy
- ◆ Social
  - ❐ social worker
  - ❐ admission to Part III, private residential, nursing home
  - ❐ Alzheimer's disease society
  - ❐ financial benefits
    attendance allowance; home help
  - ❐ incontinence nurse, district nurse
  - ❐ adaptation of home
    stickers and labels on cupboards; medicine trays
- ◆ Psychological
  - ❐ reality orientation
  - ❐ reminiscence therapy
- ◆ Support for carers
  - ❐ explanation
  - ❐ emotional support
    family/marital work; individual counselling; group; bereavement work; supportive visiting (eg. community psychiatric nurse)

- ❐ relief admissions
- ❐ introduction to voluntary sector
- ❐ practical
- ❐ financial

✱ ✱ ✱ ✱ ✱

Without doubt, a major problem for the developed world entering the new millennium is the growing number of elderly members of society. Financially, and of growing concern is how a diminishing proportion of economically active individuals can support an increasing number of non-contributors. Medically, the concern at the forefront of governing body is the increasing numbers of confused elderly, who need high levels of support.

Dementia may be considered one of the less attractive branches of medicine, but it will, inevitably, present to all doctors. Formally the province of psychogeriatricians, the confused elderly are seen by physicians for their heart and lung problems; general surgeons for their cancers; orthopaedic surgeons for their broken hips following falls; and gynaecologists. In the absence of a psychogeriatrician or, if the psychogeriatrician does not accept graduates (patients under the care of the general adult psychiatrist who reach the age of 65 years), general adult psychiatrists must deal with dementia.

Dementia is defined as an 'irreversible global deterioration in cognitive function'. If there is reversible cognitive impairment, the patient is described as suffering from an acute confusional state. But what is meant by the term 'cognitive function'? In this instance, the functions referred to include: memory, speech, visuospatial activities, personality, initiation and inhibition of action, abstract thought, calculation, recognition of objects and people. This can be summed up as mental activities that allow us to interact, in a practical sense, with the world around us. For example, if we did not have a memory, we would not know when we had sufficient to eat, or where we could find food. Visuospatial activities include functions, such as getting dressed. If this function is impaired, a person would find it confusing to put on a pair of trousers. He or she might have difficulty in working out where a leg fitted.

Such functions may be disturbed. In a young person, only a major insult, such as a severe head injury, may be necessary to affect such function. The result could be loss of memory during the time of the trauma, which may include a brief period of disorientation. However, this passes quickly, although in some cases, there may be residual disability. A more prolonged insult, such as an infection (eg. an encephalitis) over several days may have a more profound effect on functions. The person may seem less aware of his surroundings, with a lower level of consciousness. If memory fails acutely, the patient may not be able to remember where he is or what day it is, ie. disorientation in time and place. The patient may not be able to distinguish clearly what real objects are (eg. a lamp may be interpreted as a person), and may see or hear things that do not exist. Irritability, fear and agitation may follow such abnormal mental experiences. Physical factors are often easily demonstrable: infections (especially of the chest and urinary tract in the elderly); major organ failures (ie. kidney or liver); endocrine disorders (eg. hypothyroidism); factors leading to reduced oxygen supply to the brain (myocardial infarction; heart failure; anaemia) and the toxic effects of drugs, prescribed or otherwise, can all induce such a state. This usually resolves after treatment or resolution of the physical condition.

But for some people, the cognitive functions can be impaired insidiously over time, and become irreversible. Consciousness does not appear to be impaired. The first sign may be an inability to remember things, frequently the names of people with whom the sufferer is not well acquainted, and may be shrugged off as no more than can be expected with age. Such memory losses are not always indicators of disease, but if disease is present, the person may progressively fail to remember more important events and facts. The state of affairs may be confused even further if a partner or carer is present, as they may gradually take over the functions that the sufferer used to perform. Other indicators may suggest that it is more than a memory problem: the patient might start not to recognise people or objects that are familiar. He/she might not be able to dress him/herself correctly: initially buttons may be put in the wrong hole; later the patient may try to put on a pair of trousers as though they were a jumper, or put clothes on in the wrong order. The patient may become incontinent of urine or faeces; he/she could misinterpret everyday things, such as believing that the people on television are actually in the room, or may even see people who are not there. Many of these changes occur so insidiously that the partner or carer adapts without always realising anything is wrong. Sometimes, relatives mistakenly interpret effects of the illness as being due to malice on the part of the patient: it is not uncommon for a partner who does not realise the extent of the disease (or even its presence) to believe that the patient seems to forget his/her name 'on purpose'. The situation may continue until some event forces the carer to recognise that something is wrong, a psychogeriatrician is called in and the diagnosis of dementia is made.

At present, dementia is incurable, so what is the role of a psychogeriatrician? Doctors are expected to diagnose the condition, but many general practitioners have little experience of managing it, and may not even recognise it in some cases. Having diagnosed dementia, there is much that can be done. The answer is not necessarily to confine them in a nursing home or hospital. Most carers of people with dementia are close relatives (spouses, daughters or sons), and after many years of a close marriage, many carers are reluctant to accept the loss of their loved one to a home, and would rather that their spouse stayed with them, if possible, until they die. Residential care is very expensive — between £15 and £35,000 a year at 1998 prices — and either the patient or the state has to pay. Considering the number of people who develop dementia, this is not economically sustainable. So the psychogeriatrician, as part of a multi-disciplinary team that includes nurses, social workers, occupational therapists and psychologists, is involved not only in diagnosis, but also in assessment of the condition, considering how far it has advanced and what strategies might be adopted to make the situation more tolerable, allowing the carer to continue caring. For example, simple explanations about how dementia affects sufferers may help the carer to be less aggrieved by the patient's behaviour, and less reluctant to continue caring. The addition of a bath rail at home or the provision of a commode may be of practical help. Support and advice from other carers in similar situations through organisations such as the Alzheimer's Disease Society or Age Concern, may be extremely helpful. As the condition deteriorates, the patient may have to go into residential care, but he or she may have been able to spend a year or more with his/her family than might otherwise have been the case.

More specific roles for the doctor are carrying out research and detecting, investigating and treating physical illnesses (ie. chest or urinary tract infections) that may acutely aggravate the condition and which, when treated, render the situation manageable for the carer. There are many disease processes known to cause a dementing illness and researcher are trying to discover the nature of each of the processes and how they cause the cognitive impairments that are seen clinically. The main aim and hope is to find effective treatments, and much money is spent on the search for a cure. Up to the present time, such hopes have proved unfounded and new treatments have been of limited value. Progress is, however, being made and current medications, such as tacrine, donepezil and rivastigmine. are thought to have a small but significant effect on the clinical picture.

The assessment of the patient being examined for a possible dementing condition should aim to reveal the following:

- does the patient have a dementing illness?
- if the patient does have a dementing illness, to what extent?
- how much is the patient able to do for him/herself and how disabled is he/she?
- has there been a recent change (deterioration)?
- are there any reversible factors that are aggravating the situation?
- who is caring for the patient and what social support is available
- Why did the patient present now and what has led to medical help being sought?

Dementia is an irreversibly declining condition. It causes much distress. A good and thorough assessment will allow the clinician to clarify what function has irreversibly disappeared, what function might be returned and what are the current problems. Being clear about these also clarifies what needs to be done to alleviate some of the distress. The solutions may be physical, psychological (especially for the carer), educational, social or legal, or a combination of all of these. Sometimes (but not always) very simple changes can disproportionately ease the amount of distress suffered.

History of presenting complaint

The first task for the doctor is to establish the presence (or absence) of symptoms that are consistent with a diagnosis of dementia. At the early stage of the illness, the patient may be able to give symptoms; later, information will have to be obtained from informants, such as close family (spouses, adult children), neighbours or home helps. The doctor should appreciate the fact that symptoms of dementia are often not understood by relatives and friends. Difficulties with memory, praxis and personality change are often misinterpreted by others as wilful and malicious behaviour, rather than recognised as being due to illness. This is further complicated because the onset is slow in many cases —over months and years — and the first symptoms are often vague changes in personality, or mood changes, ie. Alzheimer's disease (Rubin and Kinscherf, 1989) or mild forgetfulness attributed to the ageing process. It is, therefore, important to be aware of the variety of ways such disabilities manifest in practice, for example, the patient repeatedly asks the same question. The doctor will need to question patients and carers carefully to establish the existence of symptoms that are unreported, but are causing difficulties.

There has been much debate about whether or not cognitive decline is associated with normal ageing. West *et al* suggest that there is such a decline, but that it is mild (see below). The loss of neurons that occurs with age seems to show histopathological differences from Alzheimer's disease (West *et al*, 1994). The presence of aphasia, apraxia or agnosia is thought to be a poor prognostic sign as such patients show a more rapid decline than patients with similar degree of cognitive impairment without these signs (Yesavage *et al*, 1993).

Psychotic phenomena are prominent late in dementing processes, but tend to occur as isolated phenomena (ie. part of the dementia) rather than as part of identifiable co-existent psychiatric illness (Wragg and Jeste, 1989). Hence, clinical experience is often that these symptoms do not respond to treatment with psychiatric drugs. This has additional importance, because in dementia, both verbal and physical aggressive symptoms have been regarded as related to psychotic phenomena (Aarsland *et al*, 1996). Delusions and hallucinations, symptoms of misidentification, wandering and agitation and physical aggression tend to be moderately persistent or even increase over time (Devanand *et al*, 1997).

There are many conditions that can cause a dementing process, but clinical distinction is not easy. For example, it has been suggested that vascular dementia is distinguished from Alzheimer's disease by the phenomenon of 'stepwise progression' (clear deterioration following an episode, such as a cerebrovascular accident with little change between events), but the validity of this distinction has been questioned (Zubenko, 1990). It has also been suggested that subcortical dementias, such as those due to Parkinson's disease, Huntington's disease and progressive supranuclear palsy do not show the level of apraxia, agnosia or aphasia of the cortical dementias (Huber and Paulson, 1985). It is suggested that fronto-temporal dementias show greater disinhibition, loss of personal awareness, hyperorality, perseverative behaviour and Lewy body dementia, greater complex visual hallucinations, postural instability and bradykinesia (Miller, 1997). In clinical practice, it is not unusual to find that most of these symptoms can be found in the advanced stages of dementia, whatever the aetiology.

Presentation may be precipitated by a life event, but is thought to be the social disruptiveness of change, rather than the threat implied by the life event associated with the deterioration (Orrell and Bebbington, 1995). However, the doctor should beware the clinical trap of the patient who has a comprehensible psychogenic basis to memory loss, but who, on more detailed examination and investigation (including eliciting of physical signs), is shown to have an organic basis for the process (Kopelman *et al*, 1994).

Family history

Dementia is a clinical picture that is the final common pathway in a number of conditions. Some have a significant genetic contribution (eg. Huntington's disease, which has an autosomal dominant mode of transmission); some have a significant environmental contribution (eg. dementia following head trauma, such as that seen in boxers); others have mixed, often complex contributions. Alcoholism has a genetic component (see *Chapter 1*), and alcohol abuse is known to cause dementia in a number of people. However, a number of heavy drinkers do not go on to develop dementia, suggesting an interaction of the external factor with internal predisposition. In patients with a dementing process, the relevance of the family of origin is in respect of a genetic rather than psychosocial contribution to the development of dementia.

Alzheimer's disease is the most common cause of primary dementia in the western world. It has now been established that there are different contributing factors to the development of early onset as opposed to late onset Alzheimer's disease. In early onset disease, there is an autosomal dominant transmission resulting from missense mutations in three genes: the amyloid precursor protein gene on chromosome 21 and the gene for presenilin 1 on chromosome 14 and presenilin 2 on chromosome 1. In late onset, the e4 allele of apolipoprotein E from a gene locus on chromosome 19 has been linked, although this affects when not whether the disease will manifest (Edwardson and Morris, 1998). Many other sites and associations have been proposed. There is also evidence of a genetic association between Alzheimer's disease and Down's syndrome and haematologic malignancies (Heston *et al*, 1981; Martin *et al*, 1988).

Personal history

One study found a deficiency associated with births of patients with Alzheimer's disease in May (Vezina, 1996). No such effect of season of birth was found by researchers in Australia (Henderson *et al*, 1991).

Past medical history

Many physical conditions can cause cognitive impairment, and the reader is referred to standard textbooks for the role of cardiovascular disease, neoplasia (when brain metastases are present), cerebral trauma (including boxing), infectious diseases, such as neurosyphilis, neurological disorder (eg. stroke, Parkinson's disease) and the role of impaired respiratory, hepatic, renal and endocrine (especially thyroid) function. More recently, AIDS has been recognised as a cause of dementia (Perry, 1990) and multiple sclerosis has been recognised in two patients with a clinical picture of dementia (Hotopf *et al*, 1994). Concern has increased recently about transmissible prion dementias, such as new variant Creutzfeldt-Jacob disease (Will *et al*, 1996; Fleminger and Curtis, 1997).

Past psychiatric history

There is evidence that patients with Alzheimer's disease who experience dysthymia do so in the early stages of cognitive decline, suggesting that it is a reaction to the early stages of the illness, but that major depression is experienced at all stages of dementia, with 50% of patients having a history of episodes of major depression prior to its development (Migliorelli *et al*, 1995). However, there seems to be a variant of dementia that presents initially as a late-life depression (van Ojen *et al*, 1995). Depressed mood is more common in patients with multi-infarct dementia than in Alzheimer's disease, and is less prevalent among patients with more severe Alzheimer's disease (Fischer *et al*, 1990).

There is an association between Alzheimer's disease and Down's Syndrome, but there is also evidence suggesting that others suffering from learning disabilities have a greater risk of developing dementia that increases with age, than the general population. (Cooper, 1997).

Drug history

A number of medications can cause or aggravate cognitive impairment. These include anti-cholinergic agents (Rovner *et al*, 1988), steroids (Varney *et al*, 1984) and chemotherapy used to treat cancer (Silberfarb *et al*, 1980).

Pre-morbid personality

There is evidence to suggest that there is an inverse association between smoking and Alzheimer's disease (van Duijn and Hofman, 1991), although more recent evidence questions this and suggests that smoking is a positive risk factor for Alzheimer's disease. In the case of a population studied for hypertension, cognitive decline in relation to number of cigarettes smoked occurred only in women who were of lower pre-morbid intelligence (Prince *et al*, 1996).

Social circumstances

A number of recent epidemiological studies have shown that the prevalence and incidence of dementia are increased in population strata with low compared to high levels of education. This has suggested a 'brain reserve hypothesis' in which patients with a higher level of pre-morbid intelligence, who have held jobs in which they have been in charge of subordinates, are less likely to develop dementia than those with lower pre-morbid intelligence (Schmand *et al*, 1997).

Following the suggestion that aluminium is a cause of encephalopathy in the course of renal dialysis — 'dialysis dementia' (Burks *et al*, 1976), it has been queried whether aluminium might be a cause of dementia. There is evidence that aluminosilicate is present in senile plaques in Alzheimer's disease (Candy *et al*, 1986), and it has been suggested that living in an area with high ratios of aluminium in the water could pose a risk factor for Alzheimer's disease (Rifat, 1994).

Psychosexual history

It is necessary to establish the presence or otherwise of a spouse and/or children, as these may be the carers. The willingness of the family to look after a dementing relative will be affected by the quality of the relationship prior to the onset of dementia. Despite limitation of public resources, it is not the role of professional staff to express a moral opinion, or otherwise attempt to persuade unwilling relatives to care or continue to care for a dementing patient.

Mental state examination

The mental state examination is intended to provide evidence of cognitive impairment at the time of interview, without necessarily establishing the cause. Standard tests involve testing memory and orientation, parietal and frontal lobe function as well as mood disturbance, and psychotic phenomena are described in textbooks. The use of a questionnaire, such as the Clifton Assessment Procedure of the Elderly (CAPE) or the Folstein Mini-Mental State Examination (MMSE, see below) in the clinical situation can often be helpful.

As well as clarifying the presence of cognitive impairment, the mental state examination is used to make the differential diagnosis from other psychiatric illness. Depressive illness can present a picture that can, initially, appear to be cognitive impairment: this syndrome is referred to as a depressive pseudodementia. However, there is usually other evidence of depressive illness, such as anxiety and depressive symptoms and biological symptoms of depression, such as early morning wakening or impaired libido. In contrast, patients with dementia show more disorientation and dyspraxia, such as difficulty finding their way around or impairment in tasks, such as dressing (Reynolds *et al*, 1988). Lack of insight is also qualitatively different from that found in disorders, such as schizophrenia or psychotic depression, in that denial of memory loss is inversely correlated with depressive symptoms, suggesting it may arise from disruption of the cognitive processes required for awareness of illness rather than be a defence mechanism (Sevush and Leve, 1993).

Physical examination

Patients with dementia are often thin. This may result from the underlying disease process, rather than taking inadequate nutrition (Burns *et al*, 1989).

Management

The first aspect of management is confirmation of dementia. It must be differentiated from depression, acute organic states (especially if induced by prescribed medications of which sedative and tranquillising drugs, anticholinergic drugs and antihypertensive drugs are most prominent) or alcohol abuse (Mulley, 1986).

Assessment

Clinical assessment frequently involves formal testing, such as the Folstein MMSE. There is some evidence of an association between the MMSE and cerebral atrophy found on CT scanning (Tsai and Tsuang, 1979). It is particularly useful for screening those under 20–21 years of age (MacKenzie *et al*, 1996). Cognitive function, including the MMSE, declines with age, even in the normal population. Thus, there is a risk for non-demented elderly over 85 years who have lower scores of developing dementia (Korten *et al*, 1997). The rate of decline for those over 75 years is in the order of 1.3 points/year (Brayne *et al*, 1995; Izaks *et al*, 1995). People in lower social classes (III-NM and below) and those with lower levels of education are more likely to produce lower scores than those who are in a higher social class and better educated, even when not showing evidence of cognitive decline (O'Connor *et al*, 1989). More formal cognitive testing may be carried out by neuro- psychologists.

Investigations such as CT scan and magnetic resonance imaging, especially of the temporal lobe (O'Brien *et al*, 1997), may help clinical diagnosis and differentiation from depression (O'Brien *et al*, 1994), but such investigations may not be cost effective.

Physical illness can aggravate the extent of cognitive impairment and, when it superimposes, so too can psychiatric disorder. There is evidence that treating depressive illness superimposed on dementia may improve the clinical picture of dementia (Rovner *et al*, 1989; Greenwald *et al*, 1989). Psychosocial stress can cause a pseudodelirium (Lipowski, 1983).

Aspects of management

Medication

Direct treatment

There is evidence of disturbance of many neurotransmitter systems in dementia, for example, noradrenergic and serotonergic, as well as of the neuropeptides somatostatin and CRF (Anonymous, 1987a), but on the basis that disturbance of the cholinergic system is prominent (Bowen and Davidson, 1980). The capability of anticholinergic drugs to cause disorientation and memory loss, has focussed drug treatment for Alzheimer's disease on improving cholinergic neuro-transmission. Physostigmine administered acutely intravenously improves performance on tasks of recognition memory in patients with Alzheimer's (Davis and Mohs, 1982), and has been found to be effective as an oral treatment in a few patients with Alzheimer's disease (Mohs *et al*, 1985), but there have been problems. There is evidence that newer drugs, such as tacrine, an acetylcholinesterase inhibitor, have some efficacy in retarding the progress of Alzheimer's disease (Eagger *et al*, 1991) in a small number of patients and, more recently, donepezil, a selective reversible acetylcholinesterase inhibitor, and rivastigmine have been claimed to be effective. However, therapy directed at the cholinergic system is only symptomatic rather than curative (Anonymous, 1987b).

Auxiliary medication

Management of acute behavioural disturbance, when the situation is acute or there is no easily treatable underlying cause, has involved the use of neuroleptics, such as thioridazine and haloperidol (Barnes *et al*, 1982) or benzodiazepines, such as oxazepam, and diphenhydramine. There is evidence of efficacy for all these drugs in relieving agitation in patients with dementia (Coccaro *et al*, 1990). More recently, SSRIs, such as fluoxetine (Sobin *et al*, 1989), citalopram (Nyth and Gottfries, 1990), and buspirone have been tried (Holzer *et al*, 1995). Carbamazepine has also been tried with some success (Tariot *et al*, 1998). It has been suggested that modification of the serotonergic system may be effective in demented patients who scream and bang. Greenwald *et al* (1986) suggested the use of trazodone and l-tryptophan, although an SSRI might be chosen nowadays. There is a risk of a serotonergic syndrome.

Neuroleptics are associated with sedation, extrapyramidal side-effects and a fall in blood pressure (Barnes *et al*, 1982). Some evidence suggests that use of neuroleptics may hasten cognitive decline in dementia (McShane *et al*, 1997)

Medroprogesterone acetate has been used in the management of sexually inappropriate behaviour of patients with dementia (Cooper, 1988).

Psychosocial aspects

Many patients with dementia can be managed in the community (Reifler *et al*, 1982). For some residential care will become necessary, but there is evidence to suggest that it is behavioural difficulties and psychiatric symptoms, rather than cognitive decline, that leads to institutionalisation (Steele *et al*, 1990). The ability of a patient to remain in his/her own home will depend on how far the disease has advanced, how many functions relating to self-care are satisfactorily preserved and the presence of a willing carer, usually a spouse or adult child. The patient in the early stage of disease and the carer will need information about dementia and its progression. It is also helpful to draw on the experience of previous carers in providing tips on how to deal with behaviours that give rise to distress, such as forgetting the names of spouse and children, difficulties dressing, wandering and incontinence. Help and advice is available from voluntary agencies, such as the Alzheimer's Disease Society and Age Concern in the UK. There are also booklets published by the Health Education Authority of the UK and commercially available self-help books. Brief hospitalisation can be helpful in improving behavioural problems in some patients (Zubenko *et al*, 1992).

Management of legal issues, such as informed consent, competency, powers of attorney, guardianship, inter vivos trusts, wills and living wills can ease the burden on relatives (Overman and Stoudemire, 1988). Laws vary from country to country and advice should be sought from a legally qualified practitioner. Doctors and other health and social work professionals can help their patients and carers by maintaining awareness of the major points of law in their country, but should add a suitable disclaimer about their legal expertise). In the UK, doctors should understand the concepts of power of attorney, enduring power of attorney (Dyer, 1991) and the Court of Protection. This is reviewed by Arie (1996) and Dickens (1997).

Caring for a dementing relative is extremely distressing. Doctors and other professionals involved in the care of patients with dementia should be aware of the signs of distress in carers (Goldman and Luchins, 1984; Gilleard, 1987; Morriss *et al*, 1988; Bledin *et al*, 1990; Donaldson *et al*, 1997).

Physical abuse of demented patients by their carers is a serious problem in a significant minority. Physically abusive behaviour (eg. pinching, pushing, biting, kicking, striking) is more prominent in carers who have been caring for longer, for more disabled patients, and who are experiencing depression. It is also more common in carers who were abused by the patients (Coyne *et al*, 1993).

In advising relatives of prognosis of Alzheimer's disease, Burns *et al* (1991) found that factors shown to be associated with a reduced survival over three years included: increasing age; longer duration of illness; male sex; presence of physical illnes; poor cognitive function; observed depression and absence of misidentification syndromes. Apraxia was a stronger predictor of early death than aphasia or dysmnesia.

References

Aarsland D, Cummings JL, Yenner G, Miller B (1996) Relationship of aggressive behavior to other neuropsychiatric symptoms in patients with Alzheimer's disease. *Am J Psychiatry* **153**: 243–7

Anonymous (1987a) New treatment strategies for dementia. *Lancet* **i**: 114

Anonymous. (1987b) Cholinergic treatment in Alzheimer's disease: encouraging results. *Lancet* **i**: 139–41

Arie T (1996) Some legal aspects of mental capacity. *Br Med J* **313**: 156–8

Barnes R, Veith R, Okimoto J, Raskind M, Gumbrecht G (1982) Efficacy of antipsychotic medications in behaviorally disturbed dementia patients. *Am J Psychiatry* **139**: 1170–4

Bledin KD, MacCarthy B, Kuipers L, Woods RT (1990) Daughters of people with dementia. Expressed emotion, strain and coping. *Br J Psychiatry* **157**: 221

Bowen DM, Davison AN (1980) Biochemical changes in the cholinergic system of the ageing brain and in senile dementia. *Psychol Med* **10**: 315–9

C, Gill C, Paykel ES, Huppert F, O'Connor DW (1995) Cognitive decline in an elderly population—a two wave study of change. *Psychol Med* **25**: 673–83

Burks JS, Alfrey AC, Huddleston J, Norenberg MD, Lewin E (1976) A fatal encephalopathy in chronic haemodialysis patients. *Lancet* **i**: 764–8

Burns A, Marsh A, Bender DA (1989) Dietary intake and clinical, anthropometric and biochemical indices of malnutrition in elderly demented patients and non-demented subjects. *Psychol Med* **19**: 383–91

Burns A, Lewis G, Jacoby R, Levy R (1991) Factors affecting survival in Alzheimer's disease. *Psychol Med* **21**: 363–70

Candy JM, Klinowski J, Perry RH *et al* (1986) Aluminosilicates and senile plaque formation in Alzheimer's disease. *Lancet* **I**: 354–6

Coccaro EF, Kramer E, Zemishlany Z *et al* (1990) Pharmacologic treatment of noncognitive behavioral disturbances in elderly demented patients. *Am J Psychiatry* **147**: 1640–5

Cooper AJ (1988) Medroxyprogesterone acetate as a treatment for sexual acting out in organic brain syndrome. *Am J Psychiatry* **145**: 1179–80

Cooper SA (1997) High prevalence of dementia among people with learning disabilities not attributable to Down's syndrome. *Psychol Med* **27**: 609–16

Coyne AC, Reichman WE, Berbig LJ (1993) The relationship between dementia and elder abuse. *Am J Psychiatry* **150**: 643–6

Davis , Mohs RC (1982) Enhancement of memory processes in Alzheimer's disease with multiple-dose intravenous physostigmine. *Am J Psychiatry* **139**: 1421–4

Devanand DP, Jacobs DM, Tang MX *et al* (1997) The course of psychopathologic features in mild to moderate Alzheimer disease. *Arch Gen Psychiatry* **54**: 257–63

Dickens BM)1997) Legal aspects of the dementias. *Lancet* **349**: 948–50

Donaldson C, Tarrier N, Burns A (1997) The impact of the symptoms of dementia on caregivers. *Br J Psychiatry* **170**: 62–8

Dyer C (1991) Enduring powers of attorney. *Br Med J* **303**: 77

Eagger S, Levy R, Sahakian B (1991) Tacrine in Alzheimer's disease. *Lancet* **337**: 989–92

Edwardson J, Morris C (1998) The genetics of Alzheimer's disease. *Br Med J* **317**: 361–2

Fischer P, M, Danielczyk W (1990) Depression in dementia of the Alzheimer type and in multi-infarct dementia. *Am J Psychiatry* **147**: 1484–7

Fleminger S, Curtis D (1997) Prion diseases. *Br J Psychiatry* **170**: 103–5

Gilleard CJ (1987) Influence of emotional distress among supporters on the outcome of psychogeriatric day care. *Br J Psychiatry* **150**: 219

Goldman LS, Luchins DJ (1984) Depression in the spouses of demented patients. *Am J Psychiatry* **141**: 1467–8

Greenwald BS, Marin DB, Silverman SM (1986) Serotonergic treatment of screaming and banging in dementia. *Lancet* **ii**: 1464–5

Greenwald BS, Kramer-Ginsberg E, Marin DB *et al* (1989) Dementia with coexistent major depression. *Am J Psychiatry* **146**: 1472–8

Henderson AS, Korten AE, Jorm AF, McCusker E, Creasey H, Broe GA (1991) Season of birth for Alzheimer's disease in the Southern Hemisphere. *Psychol Med* **21**: 371–4

Heston LL, Mastri AR, Anderson VE, White J (1981) Dementia of the Alzheimer type. Clinical genetics, natural history, and associated conditions. *Arch Gen Psychiatry* **38**: 1085–90

Holzer JC, Gitelman DR (1995) Price BH. Efficacy of buspirone in the treatment of dementia with aggression. *Am J Psychiatry* **152**: 812

Hotopf MH, Pollock S, Lishman WA (1994) An unusual presentation of multiple sclerosis. *Psychol Med* **24**: 525–8

Huber SJ, Paulson GW (1985) The concept of subcortical dementia. *Am J Psychiatry* **142**: 1312–7

Izaks GJ, Gussekloo J, Dermout KM, Heeren TJ, Ligthart GJ (1995) Three-year follow-up of Mini-Mental State Examination score in community residents aged 85 and over. *Psychol Med* **25**: 841–8

Kopelman MD, Green RE, Guinan EM, Lewis PD, Stanhope N (1994) The case of the amnesic intelligence officer. *Psychol Med* **24**: 1037–45

Korten AE, Henderson AS, Christensen H *et al* (1997) A prospective study of cognitive function in the elderly. *Psychol Med* **27**: 919–30

Lipowski ZJ (1983) Transient cognitive disorders (delirium, acute confusional states) in the elderly. *Am J Psychiatry* **140**: 1426–36

MacKenzie DM, Copp P, Shaw RJ, Goodwin GM (1996) Brief cognitive screening of the elderly: a comparison of the Mini-Mental State Examination (MMSE), Abbreviated Mental Test (AMT) and Mental Status Questionnaire (MSQ). *Psychol Med* **26**: 427–30

Martin RL, Gerteis G, Gabrielli WF Jr (1988) A family-genetic study of dementia of Alzheimer type. *Arch Gen Psychiatry* **45**: 894–900

McShane R, Keene J, Gedling K, Fairburn C, Jacoby R, Hope T (1997) Do neuroleptic drugs hasten cognitive decline in dementia? Prospective study with necropsy follow up. *Br Med J* **314**: 266–70

Migliorelli R, Teson A, Sabe L, Petracchi M, Leiguarda R, Starkstein SE (1995) Prevalence and correlates of dysthymia and major depression among patients with Alzheimer's disease. *Am J Psychiatry* **152**: 37–44

Miller BL (1997) Clinical advances in degenerative dementias. *Br J Psychiatry* **171**: 1–3

Mohs RC, Davis BM, Johns CA *et al* (1985) Oral physostigmine treatment of patients with Alzheimer's disease. *Am J Psychiatry* **142**: 28–33

Morris , Morris LW, Britton PG (1988) Factors affecting the emotional wellbeing of the caregivers of dementia sufferers. *Br J Psychiatry* **153**: 147

Mulley GP (1986) Differential diagnosis of dementia. *Br Med J* **292**: 1416–8

Nyth AL, Gottfries CG (1990) The clinical efficacy of citalopram in treatment of emotional disturbances in dementia. A Nordic multicentre study. *Br J Psychiatry* **157**: 894

O'Brien JT, Desmond P, Ames D, Schweitzer I, Tuckwell V, Tress B (1994) The differentiation of depression from dementia by temporal lobe magnetic resonance imaging. *Psychol Med* **24**: 633–40

O'Brien JT, Desmond P, Ames D, Schweitzer I, Chiu E, Tress B (1997) Temporal lobe magnetic resonance imaging can differentiate Alzheimer's disease from normal ageing, depression, vascular dementia and other causes of cognitive impairment. *Psychol Med* **27**: 1267–75

O'Connor DW, PA, Treasure FP, Brook CP, Reiss BB (1989) The influence of education, social class and sex on Mini-Mental State scores. *Psychol Med* **19**: 771–6

Orrell M, Bebbington P (1995) Life events and senile dementia. I. Admission, deterioration and social environment change. *Psychol Med* **25**: 373–86

Overman W Jr, Stoudemire A (1988) Guidelines for legal and financial counseling of Alzheimer's disease patients and their families. *Am J Psychiatry* **145**: 1495–500

Perry SW (1990) Organic mental disorders caused by HIV: update on early diagnosis and treatment. *Am J Psychiatry* **147**: 696–710

Prince M, Lewis G, Bird A, R, Mann A (1996) A longitudinal study of factors predicting change in cognitive test scores over time, in an older hypertensive population. *Psychol Med* **26**: 555–68

Reifler BV, Kethley A, O'Neill P, Hanley R, Lewis S, Stenchever D (1982) Five-year experience of a community outreach program for the elderly. *Am J Psychiatry* **139**: 220–3

Reynolds CF, CC, Kupfer DJ, Buysse DJ, Houck PR, Stack JA, Campbell DW (1988) Bedside differentiation of depressive pseudodementia from dementia. *Am J Psychiatry* **145**: 1099–103

Rifat SL (1994) Aluminium hypothesis lives. *Lancet* **343**: 3–4

Rovner Bwm David A, Lucas-Blaustein MJ, Conklin B, Filipp L, Tune L (1988) Self-care capacity and anticholinergic drug levels in nursing home patients. *Am J Psychiatry* **145**: 107–9

Rovner BW, Broadhead J, Spencer M, Carson K, Folstein MF (1989) Depression and Alzheimer's disease. *Am J Psychiatry* **146**: 350–3

Rubin EH, Kinscherf DA (1989) Psychopathology of very mild dementia of the Alzheimer type. *Am J Psychiatry* **146**: 1017–21

Schmand B, Smit JH, Geerlings MI, Lindeboom J (1997) The effects of intelligence and education on the development of dementia. A test of the brain reserve hypothesis. *Psychol Med* **27**: 1337–44

Sevush S, Leve N (1993) Denial of memory deficit in Alzheimer's disease. *Am J Psychiatry* **150**: 748–51

Silberfarb PM Philibert D, Levine PM (1980) Psychosocial aspects of neoplastic disease: II. Affective and cognitive effects of chemotherapy in cancer patients. *Am J Psychiatry* **137**: 597–601

Sobin P, Schneider L, McDermott H (1989) Fluoxetine in the treatment of agitated dementia. *Am J Psychiatry* **146**: 1636

Steele C, Rovner B, Chase GA, Folstein M (1990) Psychiatric symptoms and nursing home placement of patients with Alzheimer's disease. *Am J Psychiatry* **147**: 1049–51

Tariot PN, Erb R, Podgorski CA *et al* (1998) Efficacy and tolerability of carbamazepine for agitation and aggression in dementia. *Am J Psychiatry* **155**: 54-61

Tsai L, Tsuang MT (1979) The Mini-Mental State Test and computerized tomography. *Am J Psychiatry* **136**: 436–8

van Duijn CM, Hofman A (1991) Relation between nicotine intake and Alzheimer's disease. *Br Med J* **302**: 1491–4

van Ojen R, Hooijer C, Bezemer D, Jonker C, Lindeboom J, van Tilburg W (1995) Late-life depressive disorder in the community. II. The relationship between psychiatric history, MMSE and family history. *Br J Psychiatry* **166**: 316–9

Varney NR, Alexander B, MacIndoe JH (1984) Reversible steroid dementia in patients without steroid psychosis. *Am J Psychiatry* **141**: 369–72

Vezina H, Houde L, Charbonneau H *et al* (1996) Season of birth and Alzheimer's disease: a population-based study in Saguenay-Lac-St-Jean/Quebec (IMAGE Project). *Psychol Med* **26**: 143–9

West MJ, Coleman PD, Flood DG, Troncoso JC (1994) Differences in the pattern of hippocampal neuronal loss in normal ageing and Alzheimer's disease. *Lancet* **344**: 769–72

Will RG, Ironside JW, Zeidler M *et al* (1996) A new variant of Creutzfeldt-Jakob disease in the UK. *Lancet* **347**: 921–5

Wragg RE, Jeste DV (1989) Overview of depression and psychosis in Alzheimer's disease. *Am J Psychiatry* **146**: 577–87

Yesavage JA, Brooks JO, Taylor J, Tinklenberg J (1993) Development of aphasia, apraxia, and agnosia and decline in Alzheimer's disease. *Am J Psychiatry* **150**: 742–7

Zubenko GS (1990) Progression of illness in the differential diagnosis of primary dementia. *Am J Psychiatry* **147**: 435–8

Zubenko GS, Rosen J, Sweet RA, Mulsant BH, Rifai AH (1992) Impact of psychiatric hospitalization on behavioral complications of Alzheimer's disease. *Am J Psychiatry* **149**: 1484–91

Further reading

American Psychiatric Association (1997) Practice guideline for the treatment of patients with Alzheimer's disease and other of late life. *Am J Psychiatry* *154*(5 Suppl): 1–39

5

Depression

History of presenting complaint

Precipitant and/or life event

Biological symptoms

- Depressed mood with diurnal variation
- Loss of appetite
- Loss of weight
- Constipation
- Insomnia
  - ❑ initial
  - ❑ early morning wakening
- Loss of sexual interest
- Anhedonia
- Loss of concentration
- Loss of interest in things
- Feeling of lowered energy levels

Symptoms of atypical depression

- Depressed mood may be absent
- Hypersomnia
- Hyperphagia

Hypochondriacal presentation

- Problem leading to presentation
  - ❑ not eating/drinking (poor nutrition)
  - ❑ suicidal ideation

Family history

- Loss of parent
- Social class
- Physical/sexual abuse

Personal history

- Loss of job

Past medical history

- Illness associated with depression
  - ❑ cancer
  - ❑ anaemia
  - ❑ autoimmune disorder
  - ❑ cerebrovascular accident
  - ❑ hypothyroidism
  - ❑ primary
  - ❑ iatrogenic
  - ❑ uraemia
  - ❑ Addison's disease
  - ❑ Cushing's syndrome
  - ❑ severe chronic illness

Past psychiatric history

- Previous episodes of depressive illness
  - ❑ response to treatment
  - ❑ past history of treatment with antidepressants/ECT (successful or otherwise)
- Associated psychiatric disorder
  - ❑ as part of a bipolar affective disorder
  - ❑ in association with another condition
  - ❑ eating disorder
  - ❑ substance misuse
  - ❑ schizophrenia
  - ❑ dementia (with insight)

Drug history

- Drugs that can cause depression
  - ❑ corticosteroids
  - ❑ contraceptive pill (disputed)
  - ❑ cancer chemotherapy

- ❏ α-methyldopa
- ❏ H₂ antagonists
- ❏ haloperidol
- ❏ cocaine abuse (on the rebound from a high)
- ◆ Drugs being used to treat depression
  - ❏ antidepressants
  - ❏ lithium/carbamazepine

Pre-morbid personality

- ◆ Alcohol abuse

Social circumstances

- ◆ Employment
- ◆ Finances
- ◆ Relationships

Psychosexual history

- ◆ Presence of a confidant
- ◆ Marital discord/violence
- ◆ Children under the age of 11 years.

Mental state examination

Appearance

- ◆ Clothes
  - ❏ drab colours, often black; no make-up
  - ❏ poor grooming
- ◆ Evidence of failure to eat/drink
- ◆ State of the house or flat that the person lives in
  - ❏ may be very untidy or uncared for (uncharacteristically for the person)

Behaviour

- ◆ Agitation
- ◆ Psychomotor retardation
  - ❏ may be incontinent of urine or faeces

- Histrionic, dependent

Mood

- Depressed

Affect

- Downcast
    - conveying a sense of sadness
    - poor eye-contact
- Tearful

Speech

- Low volume
- Slow speech
- Long delay before replying
- Normal grammar
- 'I don't know' replies

Thoughts

- Suicidal ideation/intent/behaviour
- Paranoid ideas/delusions
- Ideas of worthlessness
- Ideas of pathological guilt
- Pessimism about the future
- Delusions
    - nihilistic

Experiences

- Mood-congruent second person auditory hallucinations
- **No** first rank symptoms

Cognition

- Picture of **pseudodementia**

Insight

- May be preserved, but often absent

Investigations

- ◆ Informant history/old case notes
- ◆ Blood tests
  - ❏ full blood count, urea and electrolytes, liver and thyroid function tests
- ◆ Research scales
  - ❏ Beck Depression Inventory
  - ❏ Hamilton Depression Rating Scale
  - ❏ Zung Depression Rating Scale
  - ❏ Hospital Anxiety and Depression Scale

Management

- ◆ Hospital admission if
  - ❏ suicidal
  - ❏ poor nutrition presenting a risk to life
- ◆ Biological treatments
  - ❏ antidepressants
    singly
      tricyclic antidepressants
      SSRIs, SNRI
      MAOIs, RIMA
      lithium
    in combination (second line therapy)
      TCA + SSRI
      TCA + Lithium
      TCA + lithium + l-tryptophan (caution)
  - ❏ ECT
- ◆ Psychotherapy
  - ❏ supportive
    counselling; cognitive-behavioural
  - ❏ dynamic
    individual
    marital
    group
- ◆ Self-help groups
  - ❏ manic-depressive fellowship

✳   ✳   ✳   ✳   ✳

An introduction to depressive illness can be found in the chapter on Hypomania

✱   ✱   ✱   ✱   ✱

History of presenting complaint

Both major psychiatric classifications (ICD-10 and DSM-IV) centre their descriptions of the clinical presentation of episodes of depressive illness around the biological symptoms of depression. Emphasis on this combination of symptoms is a common clinical experience. However, a number of different types of clinical pictures are described in the textbooks and, although they do not meet current academic criteria for a diagnosis of depressive illness, they do have a certain clinical usefulness. They include atypical depression, agitated depression, importuning dependent behaviour, peevishness in an elderly man and irritability in a younger person, somatisation or hypochondriasis, pathological grief or a pseudodementia. Nevertheless, a systematic and detailed psychopathological examination of 400 consecutive primary major depressives failed to confirm common clinical stereotypes that attribute greater somatisation, hypochondriasis, agitation, psychotic tendencies and chronicity to old age (Musetti *et al*, 1989).

Retrospective studies have consistently suggested that life events precede depressive episodes, but a recent prospective study has suggested that life events may precede non-chronic episodes of depression, but did not precede relapses in chronic unipolar or bipolar depression (Pardoen *et al*, 1996).

Family history

Family history can reveal a genetic predisposition to depressive illness or aspects of the psychosocial background, in which the patient grew up, that are known to contribute to the risk of developing depressive illness in adult life.

The prevalence of affective disorder in the first degree relatives of patients has been estimated at 10–15% compared with 1–2%in the general population (Mahmood *et al*, 1983). Twin studies of affective disorder have reported a MZ:DZ comparison of 12:0 (Essen-Moller, 1941) and 58:17 (Bertelsen, 1977) (both cited in Mahmood *et al*, 1983).

There is evidence that both a genetic contribution (as suggested by an increase MZ:DZ ratio of concordance) and shared family environment make separate and substantial contributions to the genesis of depression (McGuffin *et al*, 1991). Early loss of the mother is associated with depression (Brown *et al*, 1975 and, more recently, it has been recognised that the children of depressed parents present as clinically depressed more frequently than the children of those who are not depressed. This suggests that these children are not just experiencing a developmental phase, but are experiencing a juvenile form of depression and this may continue into adulthood (Faraone and Biederman, 1998).

In both unipolar depression and bipolar illness in childhood, there is evidence for a higher prevalence of depression, and of alcoholism and substance use disorders (Kovacs *et al*, 1997) and alcoholism in a biological parent may be a marker for depression in female offspring when compared to a background of a disturbed adoptive parent (Cadoret *et al*, 1996).

Personal history

A history of a normal psychological development from childhood and through adolescence, with satisfactory development of the personality is useful as a backdrop against which to note the change in a person who is becoming ill. A person who takes up adult responsibilities and then appears to fail to cope is suggestive of illness rather than personality difficulty and a patient who loses a job and then presents with depressive illness might have lost the job as a result of the onset of depressive illness rather than the other way around..

Long-term evidence suggests that children classified as inhibited at three years of age, and this includes children who are shy, fearful and easily upset, were more likely to meet diagnostic criteria for depression, attempt suicide and, in the case of boys, have alcohol-related problems at 21 years of age (Caspi *et al*, 1996). Adverse early experiences may predispose the person to adult depressive illness, for example, bullying, sexual or physical abuse (Pribor and Dinwiddie, 1992).

As in schizophrenia, early evidence suggests that there may be a neurodevelopmental contribution to affective disorder, especially unipolar depression. Patients with affective disorder have a higher incidence of exposure to influenza in the second trimester than controls (Machon *et al*, 1997).

Past medical history

Many illnesses have been associated with depressive illness and a list is given in *Table 5.1*. A depressive illness may present in several ways in a general medical setting:

- ◆ Depressed mood may be one symptom, and it may even indicate the presence of serious physical disease. Examples of this include: Cushing's syndrome (Mitchell and O'Keane, 1998); pancreatic carcinoma; hypothyroidis and anaemia

Table 5.1: Medical conditions associated with depressive illness

Cardiovascular	Autoimmune disorders	Surgical
◆ post myocardial infarction ◆ post CVA	◆ rheumatoid arthritis ◆ systemic lupus erythematosus ◆ temporal arteritis	◆ renal transplant ◆ coronary artery bypass graft
Endocrine disorders ◆ hypothyroidism ◆ diabetes mellitus ◆ Cushing's disease ◆ Addison's disease ◆ hypopituitarism ◆ acromegaly ◆ hypoparathyroidism ◆ hyperparathyroidism	**Infections — viral** ◆ influenza ◆ glandular ◆ herpes simplex ◆ HIV **Infections — non-viral** ◆ brucellosis ◆ typhoid	**Cancer** ◆ bronchus ◆ pancreas ◆ breast ◆ colon ◆ ovary ◆ postchemotherapy
Metabolic ◆ chronic renal failure — of itself or as a result of dialysis	**Dermatological** ◆ psoriasis ◆ eczema	**Gynaecological** ◆ post hysterectomy ◆ puerperal depression
Haematological ◆ anaemia ◆ pernicious anaemia ◆ folate deficiency	**Neurological disorders** ◆ Parkinson's disease ◆ multiple sclerosis ◆ epilepsy (especially temporal lobe)	

- several physical illnesses can cause depressive illness. This is indicated by the greater proportion of patients who become depressed when compared to other physical illnesses of equal severity. An example of this would be multiple sclerosis

- for some chronic illnesses, the process of being chronically ill can induce depression

- in other disorders, the medication given to treat the illness can cause a depressive mood change. A list of such medications is given in *Table 5.2*

- more recently, it has been appreciated that depressive illness can cause physical illness, for example, cardiovascular disease such as myocardial infarction (Musselman *et al*, 1998; Hippisley-Cox *et al*, 1998).

In some medical settings, the doctor will need to consider other options, ie. if a potential depression-inducing drug has been prescribed, the clinician should consider this in his/her the diagnosis. In medical illness, up to 50% of patients in United States studies develop clinical symptoms of depressive illnesses compared to a 6% prevalence in the general population. Depressive illness can be diagnosed in 50% of patients with a left hemispheric stroke and 10% of patients with a right hemispheric stroke; 20% of patients who have suffered a myocardial infarction (Lamberg 1996); and 24% of cancer patients (McDaniel *et al*, 1995). This ranges from 50% of those with pancreatic cancer to 1.5% of those with acute leukaemia during an admission for a bone marrow transplant. There is an increased incidence of major depression in patients with Type I diabetes mellitus compared to the general population (Popkin *et al*, 1988).

Table 5.2: Drugs thought to cause depressive mood change or illness			
Prescribed drugs		**Misused drugs**
α-methyldopa Reserpine Prednisolone Contraceptive pill ◆ especially if it contains progesterone	H₂ antagonists ◆ cimetidine, ranitidine, famotidine Haloperidol α-interferon	Crash on rebound from stimulant use ◆ cocaine, crack ◆ amphetamine CNS depressant withdrawal ◆ alcohol ◆ benzodiazepine

The seriousness of depression associated with medical conditions should not be underestimated. Renal haemodialysis, head and neck neoplasms, AIDS/HIV, SLE, renal transplantation, spinal cord injury, multiple sclerosis, peptic ulcer and malignant neoplasms are all conditions in which there is a significantly raised suicide risk (Harris and Barraclough, 1997).

Past psychiatric history

The Epidemiologic Catchment area study found a lifetime prevalence of co-morbid panic disorder of 10% in patients with unipolar depression compared with 0.8% in controls, and 20.8% in patients with bipolar disorder (Chen *et al*, 1995). The risk of recurrence of both unipolar and bipolar affective disorder is increased with the number of previous episodes (Kessing *et al*, 1998).

Alcohol dependence is a major risk factor for failure to recover from an episode of depression (Mueller *et al*, 1994) and association with major depression and/or borderline personality disorder represents a particularly high risk for suicidal symptomatology/feelings of low self-esteem, depressed alcoholics (Cornelius *et al*, 1995) and completed suicide (Lesage *et al*, 1994).

Among patients with major depressive disorder, there is a significant minority (around 25%) with social phobia or avoidant personality disorder, and two thirds have both. This latter group is more likely suffer atypical depression and greater social dysfunction than is normally expected in depressive illness (Alpert *et al*, 1997).

Pre-morbid personality

There is evidence that patients with early onset of major depression are more likely to have antecedent avoidant, histrionic, narcissistic and borderline personality disorders than those with late-onset depression (Fava *et al*, 1996b).

Recent studies have suggested that 'a certain pre-morbid personality profile — 'autonomic lability', ie. elevated neuroticism, frequent somatic complaints and increased interpersonal sensitivity — and rigidity appear to be valid antecedents of major depression' (Lauer *et al*, 1997).

Patients with major depressive disorder who have a personality disorder are likely to have a significantly worse outcome in social functioning than patients without personality disorders and are significantly more likely to have residual symptoms of depression (Shea *et al*, 1990).

Social circumstances

The absence of a confidant or low intimacy with a husband has been associated with the onset of depression (Brown *et al*, 1975). The rating of a depressed woman's relationship with her husband is predictive of her recovery from a major depressive episode (Goring *et al*, 1992). As well as with her husband, poor relationships with mother, parents-in-law, siblings and children (indicated by unruly and disobedient behaviour) are associated with episodes of depression, especially if most of the relationships are poor (Birtchnell, 1988). If a woman has a full-time job and is looking after the children, she is at increased risk of depression, and it may be precipitated by stress at work or a 'deviant' event on the part of her husband/boyfriend or child (Brown and Bifulco, 1990). For a middle-aged patient who has had an episode of major depression, the size of the social network and the subjective feeling of social support is associated with the likelihood of a relapse (George *et al*, 1989).

Conversely, there is evidence that improvement of anxiety or depression is associated with a prior positive event. In depression, feelings of a 'fresh start' — a lessening of difficulty or deprivation— is associated with improvement (Brown *et al*, 1992).

A majority of patients have work problems at the time of presentation, either through being unemployed or impaired work performance. Work outcomes are good when treatment produces symptomatic improvement, but return to work takes significantly longer than the time for symptoms to improve. In the longer term, frequent relapse is associated with poor long-term occupational outcome (Mintz *et al*, 1992).

The physical environment also affects the mood state, with depression in women on council estates associated with living in raised walkways higher than in living in tower blocks, and much higher than living in brick houses (Birtchnell *et al*, 1988).

Mental state examination

Depressed patients show objectively quantified differences from normal controls and other psychiatric patients in respect of gross motor activity, body movements, speech and motor reaction time. Psychomotor symptoms are associated with the course of illness, diurnal variation, medication status, sex and age, and are predictive of a good response to antidepressant drugs (Sobin and Sackeim, 1997).

It is important to assess for the presence of hopelessness and pessimism as there is evidence that these symptoms suggests an increased risk of suicide (Beck *et al*, 1985). Patients with unipolar depression have low self-esteem even when euthymic (Pardoen *et al*, 1993).

In respect of somatic delusions, there is a difference between the parts of the body to which the disorder is attributed, and laterality, with patients with schizophrenia localising on the left and those with affective disorder on the right (McGilchrist and Cutting, 1995).

Memory impairment in depressive illness is transient and improves with the mental state (Calev *et al*, 1986).

A recent review of mental state signs in depression suggested that the core signs for 'endogenous' depression might include: being unresponsive to the interviewer; appearing dull and inattentive; a fixed immobile face; appearing self-preoccupied; an inability to be cheered by the interviewer; slumped posture; immobility; slowed movements; slowed speech; mute or reduced speech; poverty of association; impaired insight; nihilism and observable anxiety (Parker *et al*, 1990). A paper from the same group suggests that these 'core' symptoms predict response to ECT (Hickie *et al*, 1990).

Management

The management of depression starts with proper diagnosis, but this is not as easy as it appears. Clinical experience suggests that there are patients with atypical presentations, such as those mentioned in the *History of Presenting Complaint* section of this discussion, who seem to respond to antidepressant treatment, even though it is hard to fit their symptoms and signs into the academic classifications. It is important to exclude physical illness, substance abuse, personality disorder and general dissatisfaction with life circumstances as causes of persistent low mood before making a diagnosis of primary depressive illness.

There are number of subdivisions of depressive disorder that appeared in previous classifications, but are no longer primary aspects of diagnosis. These include: unipolar/bipolar; psychotic/neurotic; endogenous/reactive. Although not part of the academic discussion, they continue to have a clinical utility. For example:

- a patient with a psychotic depression is likely to experience something analogous to a physical illness and is more likely to respond to biological treatments, whereas a patient with a neurotic depression is more likely to benefit from psychological treatments. However, it is not inappropriate to treat a patient suffering from an initial neurotic depression with an antidepressant. Many such patients obtain benefit,but the clinician must not expect the same level of response as is likely in a patient with a psychotic depression, and should avoid misdiagnosing a patient with a neurotic depression as resistant to treatment, if a response to antidepressant medication is not observed

- similarly, a patient with endogenous depression, including biological symptoms, might be considered more likely to respond to biological treatments than a patient with a reactive depression. The clinician is cautioned that some patients will develop a picture of depression with biological symptoms following a life event — the life event may be the trigger for a depressive episode to which the patient was primed.

- if a doctor is treating a patient suffering from a bipolar illness with an antidepressant drug, then the patient should be monitored more closely for signs of a manic swing. This should be followed by rapid discontinuation of the antidepressant medication (see the section on **mania** for discussion of antidepressant-induced mania).

Biological treatments, which include antidepressant medication and electroconvulsive therapy, have been demonstrated as effective in the treatment of acute depressive episodes.

- imipramine was shown to be more effective than placebo in the treatment of depressive illness in 1965 (MRC, 1965)
- monoamine oxidase inhibitors (Brandon, 1982)
- lithium was shown to be effective in the treatment of bipolar affective disorder in 1970 as a prophylactic therapy (Baastrup *et al*, 1970) and unipolar depressive disorder (Coppen *et al*, 1971).

For ethical reasons, antidepressant drugs developed in the succeeding decades have been tested against established drugs (ie. the older tricyclics) and found to be as effective, but not more so. The biological treatments have been the subject of a large literature, and an attempt will be made here to make a few salient points that are supported by research findings. For antidepressant monotherapy (ie. treatment with one antidepressant drug at a time):

- antidepressants are more likely to be helpful than psychotherapy in patients who show high social and work dysfunction and severe depressive symptoms with functional impairment (Sotsky *et al*, 1991)
- it usually takes three to four weeks for a clinical effect attributable to the drug to be observed.

It would seem that the response to an antidepressant drug is gradual, with improvement in sleep, anxiety and hostility occurring in the first week following administration of amitriptyline, and improvements occurring in the second week as steady state levels are obtained (Katz *et al*, 1991).

- antidepressant drugs have a 60–70% response rate, compared with a 30% placebo response rate, in the acute situation. The major clinical difference between the older tricyclic (TCA) and similar antidepressant drugs, and the newer generation of drugs, such as selective serotonin reuptake inhibitors (SSRI) is in the side-effect profile. In particular, there is absence of the anticholinergic side-effects of drugs, such as amitriptyline or dothiepin — although this is replaced by serotonergic side-effects, such as nausea, and some insomnia — and much higher safety in overdose. Similarly, the use of monoamine oxidase inhibitors has been limited owing to the hypertensive response to tyramine-containing food-stuffs (the 'cheese' reaction), but the development of a reversible inhibitor of monoamine oxidase makes this a strategy worth renewed consideration (Guelfi *et al*, 1992). The differences in the side-effect profile may be relevant in respect of patient compliance and important if the patient is actively suicidal, but this should not be confused with a therapeutic advance.
- a daily dose of 150mg (or its equivalent) is required for antidepressant efficacy, with some gain from doses up to 300mg (Quitkin, 1985)
- if a patient does not respond to an appropriate dose of one drug for an adequate length of time, another drug should be tried. Patients may respond idiosyncratically to one drug having failed to respond to another, but washout time must be allowed for the first drug)
- once a patient has responded to an antidepressant drug, the medication should be continued for at least six months to reduce the risk of relapse (Mindham *et al*, 1973); it has been more recently suggested that there is prophylactic benefit in continuing for five years at a daily dose of 200mg imipramine (Kupfer *et al*, 1992).

There have been reports of withdrawal symptoms with all classes of antidepressants, but patients do not experience tolerance, and so the antidepressant drugs are usually thought of as not being addictive (Young *et al*, 1997). Nevertheless, doctors should be aware that there is a street price for antidepressants (both tricyclic and SSRI), suggesting that these drugs are occasionally abused.

- there is some evidence that patients with atypical depression (according to the Columbia University criteria) respond better acutely to a MAOI, such as phenelzine, than to a TCA, such as imipramine (Liebowitz *et al*, 1988), and are maintained better after recovery by an MAOI, rather than a TCA (Stewart *et al*, 1997).

Some clinicians use lithium as an acute treatment, although there is evidence that lithium is efficacious in treating mood symptoms, but not psychosis (Goodwin *et al*, 1989). For those patients who do not respond to treatment with one antidepressant drug, there are a number of pharmacological strategies that can be tried, as appropriate:

- TCA + MAOI (Brandon, 1982; Spiker and Pugh 1976; reviews on the safety of the combination)
- TCA + SSRI (Taylor, 1995)
- TCA + Lithium (Austin *et al*, 1991)
- TCA or SSRI + lithium (Katona *et al*, 1995)
- TCA + l-tryptophan. Augmentation of antidepressant activity with tryptophan risks the eosinophilia-myalgia syndrome, so this strategy must be treated with extreme caution
- TCA + lithium + l-tryptophan (Hale *et al*, 1987).

For patients with recurrent episodes of depressive illness, prophylactic therapy should be considered.

Lithium

Lithium (as carbonate or citrate) is a toxic drug that needs to be carefully monitored. It is effective in reducing the risk of relapse (eg. Souza *et al*, 1990, unipolar depression), but if plasma levels are not carefully maintained, there is a risk of treatment failure if levels are too low and acute lithium toxicity if levels are too high. The matter is further complicated by the fact that the different commercially available lithium preparations have different pharmacokinetics. Patients are, therefore, started on low doses of lithium and plasma levels are checked at two to five days (with a t½ of around 12 hours, steady state is achieved in this time), and 11–13 hours after the last dose to see if a plasma level within the therapeutic range has been achieved. If not, the dose is increased and levels checked again two to five days later, and the process is repeated until the patient has a level in the therapeutic range. It is possible to achieve a therapeutic effect if a plasma level of 0.4–0.6 mmol/l is achieved, but treatment is more effective if the plasma level is maintained at 0.8–1.0 mmol/l (Solomon *et al*, 1996). Whether the daily dose should be given as a single dose or divided into two half-doses is disputed. Once daily dosing aids patient compliance and plasma level sampling (Coppen and Abou-Saleh, 1988). However, the potential long-term side-effects of lithium therapy include kidney and thyroid damage, although a recent review suggested that the risk of renal damage is less than originally feared (Schou, 1997). It has been suggested that it could be related to episodes of lithium intoxication rather than duration of use as a prophylaxis, and when combined with the effects of age and pre-existing renal disease may decrease renal function (Hetmar *et al*, 1991). It is uncertain whether once-daily (Plenge, 1982; Hetmar *et al*, 1991) or twice-daily (Silverstone and Turner, 1982) regimes are associated with lesser nephrotoxicity.

Hypothyroidism occurs in just under 10% of patients, but the mechanism is complex (Myers *et al*, 1985), although it has been suggested that this level may be higher, and there is some evidence that thyroid damage may be mediated through abnormalities of the immune system (Lazarus *et al*, 1981). After lithium therapy and regular checking of lithium levels has been established, renal and thyroid function should be monitored closely. Blood tests may be advised every three months. Evidence shows that setting up a regular, dedicated lithium clinic improves the technical aspects of lithium monitoring — frequency of blood tests for lithium level, renal and thyroid function — and clinical aspects — frequency and length of admission as a result of relapse (Cohen *et al*, 1993). Educational programmes for patients have been developed (Peet and Harvey, 1991). It is important that patients who are offered lithium treatment are likely to be compliant, as there is evidence that patients who discontinue lithium within the first two years have a worse clinical course than if they had not taken lithium at all (Goodwin, 1994).

There will be some patients who relapse even when taking lithium appropriately and maintaining therapeutic levels. In naturalistic follow-up studies, survival analysis data suggest that 59–73% will relapse to depressive or manic episode by five years (Gitlin *et al*, 1995; Goldberg *et al*, 1995).

After a period of stable mental health, some patients wish to discontinue lithium. Evidence suggests a slower reduction over 15–30 days is associated with a longer time to relapse than if lithium is reduced or stopped more abruptly (Baldessarini *et al*, 1997). There is also evidence that lithium is as efficacious when reinstated after relapse as it is prior to first discontinuation (Tondo *et al*, 1997). Evidence of the efficacy of lithium has recently been reviewed. Moncrieff (1995; 1997) argues that there is little evidence of efficacy in acute mania, prophylaxis of bipolar disorder and augmentation of treatment of resistant depression, but Cookson (1997) disagrees and claims that there is sufficient evidence for use in acute mania and the prophylaxis of bipolar disorder.

For patients who either do not respond to lithium, or suffer lithium toxicity, carbamazepine is a drug of second choice. There are claims that data supporting the use of carbamazepine in bipolar affective disorder are limited (Dardennes *et al*, 1995) and it is not licensed for this use in the USA, but the clinical utility of carbamazepine in this circumstance has strong advocates (Post *et al*, 1997).For patients who fail on lithium monotherapy, there is some benefit in a combination therapy of lithium plus a neuroleptic, carbamazepine or a benzodiazepine or lithium plus an antidepressant (Peselow *et al*, 1994).

Several trials have shown that electroconvulsive therapy is effective in the treatment of depressive illness. In the UK, trials have taken place at Northwick Park (Johnstone *et al*, 1980; CRC, 1984), Leicester (Brandon *et al*, 1984) and Nottingham (Gregory *et al*, 1985). West (1981) states that a convulsion is required for efficacy and 'sham' ECT — anaesthetic without administration of an electric shock — is ineffective. Twice weekly bilateral ECT is regarded as the optimum treatment. Although three treatments in a week is more effective in relieving depressive symptoms, it is associated with greater memory impairment

(Shapira *et al*, 1998). It has been claimed that patients with depressive psychosis or psychomotor retardation are most likely to respond to an acute course of ECT, but it has been suggested that among patients with a diagnosis of major depressive disorder according to RDC criteria, those patients without delusions, agitation,or psychomotor retardation were just as likely to respond acutely to a course of ECT (Sobin *et al*, 1996). ECT is an acute treatment and patients commonly relapse. Some clinicians have given maintenance ECT. Anecdotal evidence suggests this is an effective strategy and also that it does not cause deterioration in cognitive function (Barnes *et al*, 1997). ECT is sometimes effective in treatment when antidepressant medication has been ineffective. Its effect may be more obvious if the patient has been treated with an SSRI or a MAOI rather than a TCA (Prudic *et al*, 1996).

For the most refractory cases, psychosurgery has been used as a treatment. A follow-up study of stereotactic subcaudate tractotomy at six months suggested an association between improvement in psychiatric condition and a less efficient performance in certain neuropsychological tests, including verbal recognition memory, attention and two tests of frontal lobe dysfunction (Poynton *et al*, 1995).

Psychological therapies

Psychological therapies are also well established.The role of psychotherapy in the treatment of depression has been considered by Persons *et al* (1996).

Cognitive therapy

Cognitive therapy has been shown to be of benefit to patients in the acute treatment of depressive disorder in primary care (Scott *et al*, 1997) and in specialist care when maintenance cognitive therapy can have a prophylactic effect similar to antidepressant medication (Blackburn and Moore, 1997). The effect can still be observed at four year follow up (Fava *et al*, 1996a), although it should be noted that there is a relapse rate of about a third in the first year after a brief course of cognitive therapy (Thase *et al*, 1992). Predictors of response to CBT include low cognitive dysfunction (Sotsky *et al*, 1991) and although response to CBT is less than to antidepressants in severe depression (Hamilton score ≥ 20), it is still clinically significant (Thase *et al*, 1991). Cognitive therapy seems to have some advantage over imipramine in the treatment of symptoms of hopelessness and low self-esteem (Rush *et al*, 1982). There is some evidence that patients who respond to CBT have changes in the thyroid axis similar to those who respond to antidepressant treatment (Joffe *et al*, 1996), which is consistent with findings that the course of improvement in symptoms is similar for both CBT and antidepressant therapy. This suggests that improvement in cognition is due to improvement of depressive symptoms, rather than cognitive changes causing improvement in depression (Simons *et al*, 1984). It seems that in the treatment of neurotic disorder, the experience of the cognitive therapist influences the outcome (Kingdon *et al*, 1996).

Studies do not seem to support a significantly increased benefit from combination of CBT and antidepressant medication over single treatment with only one of these treatment modalities (Hollon *et al*, 1992). Notwithstanding, there is evidence that the combination of pharmacotherapy and psychotherapy do not interact negatively (Rounsaville *et al*, 1981).

Similar effects have been found for interpersonal therapy (Brown et al 1996), a brief therapy focussing on current interpersonal problems (Weissman and Markowitz, 1994). A comparison of cognitive behaviour therapy and interpersonal therapy with imipramine carried out by the National Institute of Mental Health in America was reported in 1989 (Elkin *et al*, 1989).

Evidence suggests that patients with major depression benefit from psychodynamic psychotherapy, but this is reduced if the patient has co-morbid symptoms of a personality disorder (Diguer *et al*, 1993). Bellack *et al* (1981) have shown that social skills training can be of benefit in patients with unipolar depression.

It has been suggested that, during an acute episode of depression, family pathology affects the course of depressive illness, relapse rate and suicidal behaviour. This is supported by evidence that family and marital interventions are useful in such circumstances (Keitner and Miller, 1990). When marital discord contributes to depression, O'Leary and Beach (1990) have shown that addressing it improves both depressive symptoms and marital satisfaction.

References

Alpert JE, Uebelacker LA, McLean NE *et al*, (1997) Social phobia, avoidant personality disorder and atypical depression: co-occurrence and clinical implications.*Psychol Med* **27**: 627–33

Austin MP, Souza FG, Goodwin GM (1991) Lithium augmentation in antidepressant-resistant patients. A quantitative analysis. *Br J Psychiatry* **159**: 510–14

Baastrup PC, Poulson JC Schou M, Thomsen K, Amidsen A (1970) Prophylactic lithium: double-blind discontinuation in manic depressive and recurrent depressive disorders. *Lancet* **ii**: 326–30

Baldessarini RJ, Tondo L, Floris G, Rudas N (1997) Reduced morbidity after gradual discontinuation of lithium treatment for bipolar I and II disorders: a replication study. *Am J Psychiatry* **154**: 551–3

Barnes RC, Hussein A, Anderson DN, Powell D (1997) Maintenance electroconvulsive therapy and cognitive function. *Br J Psychiatry* **170**: 285–7

Beck AT, Steer RA, M, Garrison B (1985) Hopelessness and eventual suicide: a 10-year prospective study of patients hospitalized with suicidal ideation. *Am J Psychiatry* **142**: 559–63

Bellack AS, Hersen M, Himmelhoch J (1981) Social skills training compared with pharmacotherapy and psychotherapy in the treatment of unipolar depression. *Am J Psychiatry* **138**: 1562–7

Birtchnell J (1988) Depression and family relationships: a study of young married women on a housing estate. *Br J Psychiatry* **153**: 758–69

Birtchnell J, Masters N, Deahl M (1988) Depression and the physical environment: a study of young married women on a London housing estate. *Br J Psychiatry* **153**: 56–64

Blackburn I-M, Moore RG (1997) Controlled acute and follow-up trial of cognitive therapy and pharmacotherapy in outpatients with recurrent depression. *Br J Psychiatry* **171**: 328–34

Brandon S (1982) Monoamine oxidase inhibitors in depression. *Br Med J* **285**: 1594–5

Brandon S, Cowley P, McDonald C, Neville P, Palmer R, Wellstood-Eason S (1984) Electroconvulsive therapy: results in depressive illness from the Leicestershire trial. *Br Med J* **288**: 22–5

Brown G, Ní Bhrolcháin M, Harris T (1975) Social class and psychiatric disturbance among women in an urban population. *Sociol* **9**: 225–54

Brown GW, Bifulco A (1990) Motherhood, employment and the development of depression. A replication of a finding? *Br J Psychiatry* **156**: 169–79

Brown C, Schulberg HC, Madonia MJ, Shear MK, Houck PR (1996) Treatment outcomes for primary care patients with major depression and lifetime anxiety disorders. *Am J Psychiatry* **153**: 1293–300

Cadoret RJ, Winokur G, Langbehn D, Troughton E, Yates WR, Stewart MA (1996) Depression spectrum disease, I: The role of gene-environment interaction. *Am J Psychiatry* **153**: 892–9

Calev A, Korin Y, Shapira B, Kugelmass S, Lerer B (1986) Verbal and non-verbal recall by depressed and euthymic affective patients. *Psychol Med* **16**: 789–94

Caspi A, Moffitt TE, Newman DL, Silva PA (1996) Behavioral observations at age 3 years predict adult psychiatric disorders. Longitudinal evidence from a birth cohort. *Arch Gen Psychiatry* **53**: 1033–9

Chen YW, Dilsaver SC (1995) Comorbidity of panic disorder in bipolar illness: evidence from the Epidemiologic Catchment Area Survey. *Am J Psychiatry* **152**: 280–2

Cohen RM, Douzenis A, Robinson P (1993) A lithium clinic in the real world. *Psychiatr Bull* **17**: 773

Cookson J (1997) Lithium: balancing risks and benefits. *Br J Psychiatry* **171**: 120–4

Coppen A, Noguera R, Bailey J *et al* (1971) Porphylactic lithium in affective disorders. *Lancet* **ii**: 275–9

Coppen A, Abou-Saleh MT (1988) Lithium therapy: from clinical trials to practical management. *Acta Psych Scand* **78**: 754–62

Cornelius JR, IM, Mezzich J, Cornelius MD *et al* (1995) Disproportionate suicidality in patients with comorbid major depression and alcoholism. *Am J Psychiatry* **152**: 358–64

Central Research Council (1984) The Northwick Park ECT Trial. *Br J Psychiatry* **144**: 227–37

Dardennes R, Even C, Bange F, Heim A (1995) Comparison of carbamazepine and lithium in the prophylaxis of bipolar disorders. A meta-analysis. *Br J Psychiatry* **166**: 378–81

Diguer L, Barber JP, Luborsky L (1993) Three concomitants: personality disorders, psychiatric severity, and outcome of dynamic psychotherapy of major depression. *Am J Psychiatry* **150**: 1246–8

Elkin I, Shea MT, Watkins JT *et al* (1989)National Institute of Mental Health Treatment of Depression Collaborative Research Program. General effectiveness of treatments. *Arch Gen Psychiatry* **46**: 971–82

Faraone SV, Biederman J (1998) Depression: a family affair. *Lancet* **351**: 158

Fava GA, Grandi S, Zielezny M, Rafanelli C, Canestrari R (1996a) Four-year outcome for cognitive behavioral treatment of residual symptoms in major depression. *Am J Psychiatry* **153**: 945–7

Fava M, Alpert JE, Borus JS, Nierenberg AA, Pava JA, Rosenbaum JF (1996b) Patterns of personality disorder comorbidity in early-onset versus late-onset major depression. *Am J Psychiatry* **153**: 1308–12

George LK, Blazer DG, Hughes DC, Fowler N (1989) Social support and the outcome of major depression *Br J Psychiatry* **154**: 478–85

Gitlin MJ, Swendsen J, Heller TL, Hammen C (1995) Relapse and impairment in bipolar disorder. *Am J Psychiatry* **152**: 1635–40

Goering PM, Lancee WJ, Freeman SJ (1992) Marital support and recovery from depression. *Br J Psychiatry* **160**: 76–82

Goldberg JF, Harrow M, Grossman LS (1995) Course and outcome in bipolar affective disorder: a longitudinal follow-up study. *Am J Psychiatry* **152**: 379–84

Goodwin GM, Johnson DA, McCreadie RG (1989) Comments on the Northwick Park 'Functional' Psychosis Study. *Br J Psychiatry* **154**: 406–9

Goodwin GM (1994) Recurrence of mania after lithium withdrawal. *Br J Psychiatry* **164**: 149–52

Gregory S, Shawcross CR, Gill D (1985) The Nottingham ECT Study. *Br J Psychiatry* **146**: 520–4

Guelfi JD, Payan C, Fermanian J, Pedarriosse A-M, Manfredi R (1992) Moclobemide versus clomipramine in endogenous depression. A double-blind randomised clinical trial. *Br J Psychiatry* **160**: 519–24

Hale AS, Proctor AW, Bridges PK (1987) Clomipramine, tryptophan and lithium in combination for resistant endogenous depression. *Br J Psychiatry* **151**: 213

Harris EC, Barraclough B (1997) Suicide as an outcome for mental disorders. A meta-analysis. *Br J Psychiatry* **170**: 205–28

Hetmar O, Povlsen UJ, Ladefoged J, Bolwig TG (1991) Lithium: long-term effects on the kidney. A prospective follow-up study ten years after kidney biopsy. *Br J Psychiatry* **158**: 53–8

Hickie I, Parsonage B, Parker G (1990) Prediction of response to ECT: preliminary validation of a sign-based typology of depression. *Br J Psychiatry* **157**: 65–71

Hippisley-Cox J, Fielding K, Pringle M (1998) Depression as a risk factor for ischaemic heart disease in men: population-based case-control study. *Br Med J* **316**: 1714–9

Hollon SD, DeRubeis RJ Evans MD *et al* (1992) Cognitive therapy and pharmacotherapy for depression. Singly and in combination. *Arch Gen Psychiatry* **49**: 774–81

Joffe R, Segal Z, Singer W (1996) Change in thyroid hormone levels following response to cognitive therapy for major depression. *Am J Psychiatry* **153**: 411–3

Johnstone E, Deakin JFW, Lawler P *et al* (1980) The Northwick Park ECT trial. *Lancet* **ii**: 1317–20

Katona CLE, Abou-Saleh MT, Harrison DA *et al* (1995) Placebo-controlled trial of lithium augmentation of fluoxetine and lofepramine. *Br J Psychiatry* **166**: 80–6

Katz MM, Koslow SH, Maas JW *et al* (1991) Identifying the specific clinical actions of amitriptyline: interrelationships of behaviour, affect and plasma levels in depression. *Psychol Med* **21**(3): 599–611

Keitner GI, Miller IW (1990) Family functioning and major depression: an overview. *Am J Psychiatry* **147**(9): 1128–37

Kessing LV, Andersen PK, Mortensen PB, Bolwig TG (1998) Recurrence in affective disorder. I. Case register study. *Br J Psychiatry* **172**: 23–8

Kingdon D, Tyrer P, Sievewright N, Ferguson B, Murphy S (1996) The Nottingham study of neurotic disorder: influence of cognitive therapists on outcome. *Br J Psychiatry* **169**: 93–7

Kovacs M, Devlin B, Pollock M, Richards C, Mukerji P (1997) A controlled family history study of childhood-onset depressive disorder. *Arch Gen Psychiatry* **54**: 613–23

Kupfer DJ, Frank E, Perel JM *et al* (1992) Five-year outcome for maintenance therapies in recurrent depression. *Arch Gen Psychiatry* **49**(10): 769–73

Lamberg L (1996) Treating depression in medical conditions may improve quality of life. *JAMA* **276**: 857–8

Lauer CJ, Bronisch T, Kainz M, Schreiber W, Holsboer F, Krieg JC (1997) Pre-morbid psychometric profile of subjects at high familial risk for affective disorder. *Psychol Med* **27**(2): 355–62

Lazarus JH, John R, Bennie EH, Chalmers RJ, Crockett G (1981) Lithium therapy and thyroid function: a long-term study. *Psychol Med* **11**(1): 85–92

Lesage AD, Boyer R, Grunberg F *et al* (1994) Suicide and mental disorders: a case-control study of young men. *Am J Psychiatry* **151**(7): 1063–8

Liebowitz MR, Quitkin FM, Stewart JW *et al* (1988) Antidepressant specificity in atypical depression. *Arch Gen Psychiatry* **45**(2): 129–37

Machon RA, Mednick SA, Huttunen MO (1997) Adult major affective disorder after prenatal exposure to an influenza epidemic. *Arch Gen Psychiatry* **54**: 322–8

Mahmood T, Reveley AM, Murray RM (1983) Genetic studies of affective and anxiety disorders. In: Weller M, ed. *The Scientific Basis of Psychiatry*. Balliere Tindall, London

McDaniel JS, Musselman DL, Porter MR, Reed DA, Nemeroff CB (1995) Depression in patients with cancer. Diagnosis, biology and treatment. *Arch Gen Psychiatry*. **52**: 89–99

McGilchrist I, Cutting J (1995) Somatic delusions in schizophrenia and the affective psychoses. *Br J Psychiatry* **167**(3): 350–61

McGuffin P, Katz R, Rutherford J (1991) Nature, nurture and depression: a twin study. *Psychol Med* **21**(2): 329–35

Medical Research Council (1965) Clinical Medical Research Council. Clinical trial of the treatment of depressive illness. *Br Med J* i: 8816–

Mindham R, Howland C, Shepherd M (1973) An evaluation of continuation therapy with tricyclic antidepressants in depressive illness. *Psychol Med* **3**: 5–17

Mintz J, Mintz LI, Arruda MJ, Hwang SS (1992) Treatments of depression and the functional capacity to work. *Arch Gen Psychiatry* **49**(10): 761–8

Mitchell A, O'Keane V (1995) Steroids and depression. *Br Med J* 1998;316:244-5 nation of the placebo-controlled trials of lithium prophylaxis in manic depressive disorder. *Br J Psychiatry* **167**: 569–73

Moncrieff J (1997) Lithium: evidence reconsidered. *Br J Psychiatry* **171**: 113–9

Mueller TI, Lavori PW, Keller MB *et al* (1994) Prognostic effect of the variable course of alcoholism on the 10-year course of depression. *Am J Psychiatry* **151**(5): 701–6

Musetti L, Perugi G, Soriani A, Rossi VM, Cassano GB, Akiskal HS (1989) Depression before and after age 65. A re-examination. *Br J Psychiatry* **155**: 330–6

Musselman DL, Evans DL, Nemeroff CB (1998) The relationship of depression to cardiovascular disease: epidemiology, biology, and treatment. *Arch Gen Psychiatry* **55**: 580–92

Myers DH, Carter RA, Burns BH, Armond A, Hussain SB, Chengapa VK (1985) A prospective study of the effects of lithium on thyroid function and on the prevalence of antithyroid antibodies. *Psychol Med* **15**(1): 55–61

O'Leary KD, Beach SR (1990) Marital therapy: a viable treatment for depression and marital discord. *Am J Psychiatry* **147**: 183–6

Pardoen D, Bauwens F, Tracy A, Martin F, Mendlewicz J (1993) Self-esteem in recovered bipolar and unipolar out-patients. *Br J Psychiatry* **163**: 755–62

Pardoen D, Bauwens F, Dramaix M *et al* (1996) Life events and primary affective disorders. A one year prospective study. *Br J Psychiatry* **169**: 160–6

Parker G, Hadzi-Pavlovic D, Boyce P *et al* (1990) Classifying depression by mental state signs. *Br J Psychiatry* **157**: 55

Peet M, Harvey NS (1991) Lithium maintenance: 1. A standard education programme for patients. *Br J Psychiatry* **158**: 197–200

Persons JB, Thase ME, Crits-Christoph P (1996) The role of psychotherapy in the treatment of depression: review of two practice guidelines. *Arch Gen Psychiatry* **53**(4): 283–90

Peselow ED, Fieve RR, Difiglia C, Sanfilipo MP (1994) Lithium prophylaxis of bipolar illness. The value of combination treatment. *Br J Psychiatry* **164**(2): 208–14

Plenge P, Mellerup ET, Bolwig TG *et al* (1982) Lithium treatment: does the kidney prefer one daily dose instead of two? *Acta Psych Scand* **66**: 121–8

Popkin MK, Callies AL, Lentz RD, Colon EA, Sutherland DE (1988) Prevalence of major depression, simple phobia, and other psychiatric disorders in patients with long-standing type I diabetes mellitus. *Arch Gen Psychiatry* **45**(1): 64–8

Post RM, Denicoff KD, Frye MA, Leverich GS (1997) Re-evaluating carbamazepine prophylaxis in bipolar disorder. *Br J Psychiatry* **170**: 202–4

Poynton AM, Kartsounis LD, Bridges PK (1995) A prospective clinical study of stereotactic subcaudate tractotomy. *Psychol Med* **25**(4): 763–70

Pribor EF, Dinwiddie SH (1992) Psychiatric correlates of incest in childhood. *Am J Psychiatry* **149**(1): 52–6

Prudic J, Haskett RF, Mulsant B *et al* (1996) Resistance to antidepressant medications and short-term clinical response to ECT. *Am J Psychiatry* **153**: 985–92

Quitkin FM (1985) The importance of dosage in prescribing antidepressants. *Br J Psychiatry* **147**: 593–7

Rounsaville BJ, Klerman Gl, Weissman MM (1981) Do psychotherapy and pharmacotherapy for depression conflict? Empirical evidence from a clinical trial. *Arch Gen Psychiatry* **38**(1): 24–9

Rush AJ, Beck AT, Kovacs M, Weissenburger J, Hollon SD (1982) Comparison of the effects of cognitive therapy and pharmacotherapy on hopelessness and self-concept. *Am J Psychiatry* **139**(7): 862–6

Schou M (1997) Forty years of lithium treatment. *Arch Gen Psychiatry* **54**: 9–13

Scott C, Tacchi MJ, Jones R, Scott J (1997) Acute and one-year outcome of a randomised controlled trial of brief cognitive therapy for major depressive disorder in primary care. *Br J Psychiatry* **171**: 131 4

Shapira B, Tubi N, Drexler H, Lidsky D, Calev A, Lerer B (1998) Cost and benefit in choice of ECT schedule. Twice weekly versus three times weekly ECT. *Br J Psychiatry* **172**: 44–8

Shea MT, Pilkonis PA, Beckham E *et al* (1990) Personality disorders and treatment outcome in the NIMH Treatment of Depression Collaborative Research Program. *Am J Psychiatry* **147**(6): 711–8

Silverstone T,Turner P (1982) *Drug Treatment in Psychiatry*. Routledge,Kegan and Paul, London

Simons AD, Garfield SL, Murphy GE (1984) The process of change in cognitive therapy and pharmacotherapy for depression. Changes in mood and cognition. *Arch Gen Psychiatry* **41**(1): 45–51

Sobin C, Prudic J, Devanand DP, Nobler MS, Sackeim HA (1996) Who responds to electroconvulsive therapy? A comparison of effective and ineffective forms of treatment. *Br J Psychiatry* **169**: 322–8

Sobin C, Sackeim HA (1997) Psychomotor symptoms of depression. *Am J Psychiatry* **154**: 4–17

Solomon DA, Ristow WR, Keller MB *et al*)1996) Serum lithium levels and psychosocial function in patients with Bipolar I Disorder. *Am J Psychiatry* **153**: 1301–7

Sotsky SM, Glass DR, Shea MT *et al* (1991) Patient predictors of response to psychotherapy and pharmacotherapy: findings in the NIMH Treatment of Depression Collaborative Research Program. *Am J Psychiatry* **148**: 997–1008

Souza FG, Mander AJ, Goodwin GM (1990) The efficacy of lithium in prophylaxis of unipolar depression Evidence from its discontinuation. *Br J Psychiatry* **157**: 718–22

Spiker DG, Pugh DD (1976) Combining tricyclic and monoamine oxidase inhibitor antidepressants. *Arch Gen Psychiatry* **33**: 828–30

Stewart JW, Tricamo E, McGrath PJ, Quitkin FM (1997) Prophylactic efficacy of phenelzine and imipramine in chronic atypical depression: likelihood of recurrence on discontinuation after 6 months' remission. *Am J Psychiatry* **154**: 31–6

Taylor D (1995) Selective serotonin reuptake inhibitors and tricyclic antidepressants in combination. Interactions and therapeutic uses. *Br J Psychiatry* **167**: 575

Thase ME, Simons AD, Cahalane J, McGeary J, Harden T (1991) Severity of depression and response to cognitive behavior therapy. *Am J Psychiatry* **148**(6): 784–9

Thase ME, Simons AD, McGeary J *et al* (1992) Relapse after cognitive behavior therapy of depression: potential implications for longer courses of treatment. *Am J Psychiatry* **149**: 1046–52

Tondo L, Baldessarini RJ, Floris G, Rudas N (1997) Effectiveness of restarting lithium treatment after its discontinuation in bipolar I and bipolar II disorders. *Am J Psychiatry* **154**(4): 548–50

Weissman MM, Markowitz JC (1994) Interpersonal psychotherapy. Current status. *Arch Gen Psychiatry* **51**(8): 599–606

West ED (1981) Electric convulsion therapy in depression a double-blind controlled trial. *Br Med J* **282**: 355–7

Young AH, Currie A, Ashton CH (1997) Antidepressant withdrawal syndrome. *Br J Psychiatry* **170**: 288

Further reading

Hirschfield RMA, Clayton, Cohen I *et al* (1994) American Psychiatric Association Guidelines for Bipolar Disorder. *Am J Psychiatry* 151(Suppl): S1–S36

6

Hypomania

History of presenting complaint

Precipitant to episode and/or life event

- ◆ Symptoms
  - ❑ elated mood
  - ❑ disinhibition
    socially and sexually
  - ❑ spending money
  - ❑ grandiose plans
  - ❑ inability to concentrate on one line of thought
  - ❑ increased volubility
  - ❑ insomnia
    especially secondary to 'not having enough time to get everything done'
  - ❑ irritability
  - ❑ overactivity, restlessness
  - ❑ feeling of increased energy
  - ❑ increased alcohol intake (at times of elevated mood only)
  - ❑ mood-congruent delusions and hallucinations
- ◆ Problem leading to presentation

Family history

- ◆ Family history of hypomania

Personal history

- ◆ Loss of job
  - ❑ episodes of interruption of work record, but return to previous level of functioning between episodes

Past medical history

- ◆ Illnesses associated with hypomania
    - ❏ thyrotoxicosis
    - ❏ autoimmune disorders
    - ❏ Cushing's syndrome
- ◆ Treatments causing hypomania
    - ❏ thyroxine treatment for hypothyroidism
    - ❏ steroid replacement therapy

Past psychiatric history

- ◆ Previous episodes of hypomania
- ◆ Associated psychiatric illness
    - ❏ depression as part of a bipolar illness
    - ❏ schizophrenia
    - ❏ early dementia
    - ❏ drug abuse

        stimulants: cocaine, amphetamine; hallucinogens (LSD)
        procyclidine

Drug history

- ◆ Drugs for treatment of physical illness
    - ❏ thyroxine
    - ❏ corticosteroids
    - ❏ H_2 antagonists

        cimetidine
        ranitidine
        famotidine
- ◆ Drugs for treatment of psychiatric illness
    - ❏ that might have precipitated hypomania

        antidepressant drugs
    - ❏ that might have been prescribed for the treatment of hypomania

        lithium
        carbamazepine
        sodium valproate

Pre-morbid personality

- Normal personality when not hypomanic
- Religious beliefs to ascertain cultural background of any beliefs

Forensic history

- Illicit drug use

Social circumstances

- Ownership of property
- Extent of family and whether still supportive

Psychosexual history

Often patients are established in a satisfactory relationship prior to first episode of hypomania:

- Nature of current relationship
- Extent of incongruity of any disinhibited behaviour with relationships when well

Mental state examination

Appearance

- Clothing
  - bright colours
  - significant objects tallying with grandiose ideas
- Make-up
  - lipstick

    often applied slightly inaccurately round the mouth
    bright in colour

Behaviour

- Posture may be grandiose; eg. manic stupor ('beatification')
- Overactive or restless
  - the patient may not be able to sit down throughout the interview and is constantly on the move
- Patient may be inebriated

Mood

- Happy, usually excessively so

Affect

- Euphoric, giggling, infectious good humour
- Easily irritated if frustrated
- Irritable
- May give that impression that she/he is unhappy under the surface (manic defence)

Speech

- Pressure of speech
- Flight of ideas
- Loud volume

Thoughts

- Excessive optimism
- Unrealistic plans
- Paranoid ideas
- Inflated self-esteem
- Grandiose delusions

Experiences

- Second person auditory hallucinations, mood-congruent
- First rank symptoms may be present

Cognition

- Intact

Insight

- Absent

Investigations

- Urine drug screen

Management

- Hospital admission
  - ❑ may need compulsory admission

Stop antidepressants, thyroxine or other drugs that precipitate elevated mood

- ◆ Drug treatment
  - ❏ neuroleptics acutely
  - ❏ lithium, carbamazepine, sodium valproate can be used as longer-term treatment
- ◆ Outpatient follow-up
  - ❏ monitoring of mental state and early detection of relapse
  - ❏ monitoring of lithium
    regular estimation of lithium level
    detection of clinical symptoms indicative of toxicity
    regular monitoring of renal and thyroid function
- ◆ Self-help groups
  - ❏ manic-depressive fellowship

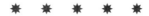

Imagine a time that something really good happened. Not just something nice, but something really good. Your partner proposed. You got your new car. You saw that you had passed your exams. You name it, but it was good. How did you feel when it happened? Happy, perhaps. You felt like going out and doing things. Great plans came into your head. You felt like laughing, and wanted all the world to join in. You felt like being silly, perhaps playing a practical joke on someone: or at least cracking a lot of jokes. You felt like having a drink, a party, dressing up and going out.

But the next day, after a late night, and perhaps nursing a hangover — 'I'll never get drunk like that again,' you say — you come down to earth. You are still happy, but not excessively so. You recognise that you have been euphoric, and that the mood is settling. Life returns to normal.

For some people, such euphoric moods can develop without a precipitating factor. They can be happy, giggling, constantly talking, making jokes and puns. They induce humour in those around them. They have lots of ideas, and may act on them, even if they are unwise. They might spend money more freely than is wise and end up in financial difficulties. They may be sexually disinhibited. If their ideas and plans are interfered with, they become easily irritated. The euphoria lasts not just a few hours, but days, weeks and even months. This is not just normal high spirits, and psychiatrists recognise it as an illness — hypomania. Some people in this state can hear voices, often talking to them, telling them how wonderful they are; and they can come to believe that they are particularly important or have a particularly important mission (in England, it is not uncommon to find people with hypomania who believe that they are Jesus Christ).

In the acute situation, patients with hypomania often cannot be nursed at home and hospital admission, not infrequently compulsorily under a section of the Mental Health Act 1983, is necessary. There, acute treatment is with neuroleptics, and although there is little or no evidence for its use, haloperidol is the fashionable neuroleptic in hypomania. Perhaps the fact that it can be given intramuscularly or intravenously to a disturbed patient boosts its popularity. Patients in this situation often settle down after about two or three weeks.

At the other end of the spectrum is depressed mood. This is not the opposite of elation as there are patients who exhibit both types of symptoms simultaneously ('mixed affective state'). This suggests that the neural mechanisms control independent systems. These may have a mechanism for reciprocal inhibition that has failed. The feeling of depression is familiar and is common after receiving bad news. As well as feeling unhappy and perhaps crying, a person may not feel like doing anything; favourite programmes are no longer of interest (the avid fan may not be interested in 'Neighbours' or their other favourite soap that evening!) and he or she is disinclined to eat. Sleep may not come easily. Things that at other times assume great importance seem very trivial and other people's anxieties seem insignificant and irritating. Indeed the person may not want to be with other people and wishes to be left alone. There may seem no point to anything, even life.

But, as with elation, the depressed mood eases after a few hours, and 'things' are once again seen in perspective. However, those who continue in such a mood state for an extended period are diagnosed as suffering from an illness. They may stop eating or drinking for so long that there is a serious risk to life, or they could attempt suicide. Such an attempt should not be regarded as just a 'cry for help'. Some may hear voices telling them how awful they are, develop abnormal beliefs (delusions) that they are dead or have incurable cancer. They may even imagine they have committed crimes that deserve severe punishment quite out of proportion to the alleged crimes, such as the death penalty for giving another person a penny too little change 30 years ago. Thus, the term **depressive illness** covers a spectrum from the mildly depressed to the most severely ill. The **biological symptoms of depression** include: depressed mood, with diurnal variation; insomnia, with early morning wakening; loss of appetite; loss of weight and severe constipation; loss of libido (loss of interest in sex); loss of ability to gain pleasure from things (**anhedonia**) and loss of concentration. It has been suggested that the presence of biological symptoms is a favourable indication of patients who are likely to respond to tricyclic antidepressants.

In addition, if the diagnosis of depression is that severity and duration characterise the difference between depressed mood and depressive illness, where should we draw the line? In patients where the severity of the illness needs psychiatric treatment from a consultant, diagnosis is often easy; definition is much harder in general practice. If mood varies in response to external events, and if a person is encountering numerous negative experiences in his or her daily life, when is it depression? For example, a woman in her late 20s with three young children, all under five years of age. Her husband is often out, either at work or at the pub. He does not pay the bills, but expects his food to be on the table. She has a part-time job, but the money is not enough. The children are demanding. She keeps the flat they live in tidy, but if there is one speck of dust, her husband criticises her mercilessly. Week after week she complains of depressed mood, refusing to acknowledge that re-adjusting her relationship with her husband might help, and her mood varies according to whether he shouted at her this week. She wants a pill for her depression. Is she depressed? Will an antidepressant help?

Technically, depression has been defined in various unsatisfactory ways: neurotic versus psychotic depression (ie. depression with or without psychosis); endogenous versus reactive (ie. occurring spontaneously compared with depression arising in response to an external event); unipolar versus bipolar (ie. episodes of depression alone or episodes of depression interspersed with episodes of hypomania). Such distinctions may represent clinical presentations, but have not been shown to be of value in aetiology or treatment.

What is clear is the number of patients who suffer from recurrent episodes of mood disorder that includes episodes of hypomania and depression. The changes between hypomania and depression are described as mood swings, and since the 1950s, lithium has been used for the treatment of bipolar affective disorder. It is possible to use lithium in the acute situation, but it still takes a week or more to be effective, and so it tends not to be used for a newly admitted hypomanic patient who is very disturbed. The tranquillising effect of neuroleptics is more useful in the acute situation.

Lithium is the drug of choice in prophylactic use. Studies have shown that it reduces the frequency and intensity of mood swings and if a patient has a second episode of affective disorder, the clinician will want to consider using lithium. However, it is not without problems. Lithium is a very toxic drug and in excessive doses, in the plasma, it can be fatal; in inadequate dosage it is ineffective. It is, therefore, a drug that requires close monitoring and psychiatrists and GPs who wish to treat their patients for bipolar affective disorder need to know how to do this.

The main, long-term risks of lithium therapy are damage to the kidney and the thyroid, with the risk that hypothyroidism may precipitate depression and could aggravate or induce the condition it is supposed to alleviate. Thus, as well as monitoring the level of lithium in the blood, renal and thyroid function should be monitored closely. When instituting lithium therapy, renal and thyroid function tests should be carried out prior to treatment. If these are satisfactory, lithium should be gradually introduced. The doctor should start with a low dose (eg. 400mg daily) and blood levels should be taken at 11–13 hours after the last dose approximately two to five days after starting at that dose. If the resulting level is shown to be in the therapeutic range, then the patient should continue to take that dose. Should the level be too low, the total daily dose should be increased by 200mg, and the test repeated two to five days later. This cycle should be repeated until the patient has a level in the therapeutic range. Initial weekly checks should ensure that the patient is stable on this dose. Once stabilised, regular checks of lithium level and renal and thyroid function should be made. In general, a patient should remain on lithium for at least five years. Attempts to stop medication can then be tried, but patients have been known to relapse after being symptoms free throughout the five years. It is difficult to return the patient to the clinical state they were in before stopping lithium.

In countries where plasma level monitoring of lithium and anticonvulsants is not readily available, or for patients who are unwilling to co-operate with blood tests, it may be imprudent to prescribe lithium or carbamazepine. Chronic neuroleptic therapy is regarded as a possible, but second-line, prophylactic therapy for bipolar affective disorder. As for other disorders where chronic neuroleptic therapy is used, a depot preparation can be a useful mode of administration.

* * * * *

History of presenting complaint

The symptoms of hypomania are essentially undisputed. Different combinations of clinical presentation seem to be possible, with at least one variant in which dysphoric symptoms are mixed with the symptoms of elated mood (Cassidy *et al*, 1998). There has been interest in precipitants to hypomanic episodes, including sleep deprivation (Wright, 1993) and seasonal variation and life events. There is a recognisable seasonal pattern to the onset of hypomania in a significant minority of patients with bipolar disorder (Carney *et al*, 1988). There are two patterns: (a) winter depression ± summer hypomania and (b) summer depression ± winter hypomania (Faedda *et al*, 1993).

There is some uncertainty about whether life events can precipitate episodes of hypomania. Evidence suggests that life events can precipitate episodes (Hammen and Gitlin, 1997), especially if these events are threatening (Chung *et al*, 1986), although this has not always been found (Sclare and Creed, 1990). There is some suggestion that the effect of life events is only found in early episodes of the mania (McPherson *et al*, 1993).

Presentation of a first manic episode in an elderly person is suggestive of an underlying organic cerebral impairment (Stone, 1989), an associated neurological disorder (Tohen *et al*, 1994), or other cerebral insult (Snowdon, 1991). Compliance with medication and shorter duration of illness have been associated with recovery from an episode of hypomania (Keck *et al, 1998)*.

Family history

The genetic contribution to affective disorder is complicated and has not been clarified. It has been suggested that the familial aggregation of bipolar disorder may have a genetic factor (McGuffin and Katz, 1989). Recent studies show that patients with early onset affective psychosis are more likely to have a family history of affective disorder or substance abuse disorder than patients with late onset (Sax *et al*, 1997; Stone, 1989).

Patients with bipolar I disorder have an increased family history of mania compared to both patients who have unipolar depression and controls (Winokur *et al*, 1995b). Kendler *et al* (1993) found a concordance rate of 48.2% in MZ and 23.4% in DZ twins for affective illness by DSM-IIIR criteria. There seems to be a greater incidence of unipolar and bipolar illnesses breeding true, but this is not always the case. There has been considerable research for a molecular genetic basis for this and several genes and chromosomes have been examined, including:

- possible linkage tyrosine hydroxylase, tyrosinase, and D2 and D4 dopamine receptor genes on chromosome 11 (Smyth *et al*, 1996; De Bruyn *et al*, 1994)
- a susceptibility gene near the centromere of chromosome 18 (Berrettini *et al*, 1997)
- deleted short arm of chromosome 21 (el-Badramany *et al*, 1989)
- an association between velo-cardio-facial syndrome and early-onset bipolar disorder with suggestion of a gene deletion at the 22q11 chromosomal locus (Papolos *et al*, 1996)
- the X-chromosome (Berrettini *et al*, 1990; Mendlewicz, 1992; Hebebrand 1992)
- an association with the tryptophan hydroxylase gene (Bellivier *et al*, 1998)

- the dopamine (D2) receptor gene (Holmes *et al*, 1991)
- the COMT gene (Gutierrez *et al*, 1997)
- gene for the G protein stimulatory alpha subunit (Ram *et al*, 1997)
- thalassaemia minor (Singh and Maguire, 1988).

Personal history

There is evidence that a patient's affective disorder may have a history of neurodevelopmental impairment (van Os *et al*, 1997), low educational test scores, late attainment of motor milestones, speech defects between 6 and 15, decreased psychomotor alertness on medical examination between 4 and 11 and an excess of twitching and grimacing motor behaviours in adolescence. Patients with bipolar disorder often have a history of poor social functioning in adolescence but function well at school (Cannon *et al*, 1997).

Past medical history

Hypomania has been reported as a secondary complication of a number of medical conditions, including:

- AIDS (Dauncey, 1988; Schmidt, 1988; Lyketsos *et al*, 1993) as a prelude to AIDS dementia, and as a complication of treatment with didanosine (Brouillette *et al*, 1994)
- B12 deficiency (Goggans, 1984)
- Cardiovascular disease
  - cardiac arrest (Kumar and Agarwal, 1988)
  - after open heart surgery (Isles and Orrell, 1991)
- Cerebrovascular lesions: subarachnoid haemorrhage (Jampala and Abrams, 1983; Cummings and Mendez, 1984; Starkstein and Robinson, 1989; Blackwell, 1991); left basal-ganglia stroke (Berthier, 1992; Turecki *et al*, 1993)
- Cushing's syndrome (Haskett, 1985)
- Meningeal *cryptococcosis* (Thienhaus and Khosla, 1984)
- Epilepsy: complex partial seizures (Barczak *et al*, 1988) temporal lobe damage; (Byrne, 1988; Johnson and Campbell, 1990); primary generalised epilepsy (Howland, 1993)
- Haematological disorder
  - polycythaemia rubra vera (Chawla and Lindesay, 1993)
  - Christmas disease (Gill *et al*, 1992; Craddock and Owen, 1992)
- Head injury (Shukla *et al*, 1987; Bracken, 1987; Bell *et al*, 1987; Clark and Davison, 1987; Yatham 1987; McKeown and Jani, 1987; Robinson *et al*, 1988; Bamrah and Johnson, 1991; Jorge *et al*, 1993; Collins and Jacobson, 1990); anoxic brain damage (Calache and Bourgeois, 1990)
- Kidney disease (Wylie *et al*, 1993)
- Multiple sclerosis (Buckley and Hutchinson, 1993)
- Normal pressure hydrocephalus (Schneider *et al*, 1996)

- sarcoidosis (Walbridge, 1990; McLoughlin and McKeon, 1991)
- Thyrotoxicosis (Lee *et al*, 1991); hypothyroidism is associated with rapid cycling (Bauer *et al*, 1990)
- Urticaria (Harvey and Mikhail, 1986)
- Uraemia (Thomas and Neale, 1991; Benazzi, 1991).

Past psychiatric history

The course of bipolar affective disorder is not always benign and the risk of further episodes and admissions is increased for greater numbers of previous admissions and episodes (Joyce, 1985, Kessing *et al*, 1998). There is evidence of increased co-morbidity with panic disorder in patients with bipolar illness, greater than for unipolar depression (Chen *et al*, 1995) and it has been suggested that there is a degree of co-morbidity of mania with personality disorder (Peselow *et al*, 1995), with evidence of personality disorder even when the patient is euthymic.

The situation with alcohol is complicated, as the direction of morbidity goes in both directions. There is some evidence that alcoholism can be secondary to hypomania (Winokur *et al*, 1995a). This complicates the clinical picture as substance misuse is inversely correlated with recovery from the manic or mixed affective episode (Keck *et al*, 1998) and co-morbid substance misuse and medication non-compliance were suggested as the most important factors contributing to rehospitalisation of patients with schizophrenic, schizoaffective, and affective disorders (O'Connell *et al*, 1991; Haywood *et al*, 1995; Strakowski *et al*, 1998).

Drug history

A number of medications (or their withdrawal) can precipitate manic episodes and should be investigated. Antidepressant drugs can precipitate mania. Incidence has been reported as 2.6–35% (Kupfer *et al*, 1988; Altshuler *et al*, 1995). The effect is not specific to any one drug or group of drugs, and there have been reports of antidepressant-induced hypomania with mianserin (Sturdy and Mahapatra, 1988); MAOIs (Pickar *et al*, 1982) or augmented with l-tryptophan (Goff, 1985); lithium augmentation (Yuvarajan and Yousufzai, 1988); paroxetine (Christensen, 1995), fluoxetine (Steiner, 1991, Berthier and Kulisevsky, 1993), citalopram (Bryois and Ferrero, 1994), sertraline (Laporta, 1987); trazodone (Zmitek, 1987; Jabeen and Fisher, 1991), nefazodone (Dubin *et al*, 1997). There is some evidence that when antidepressants induce a manic episode, the illness is less severe and lasts for a shorter duration than when the manic episode arises spontaneously (Stoll *et al*, 1994). It should be noted that there is a possibility that ECT can induce a manic episode (Sanders and Deshpande, 1990).

Withdrawal of mood-stabilising medication, such as lithium (Harrison-Read, 1998) or carbamazepine (Scull and Trimble, 1995) can precipitate hypomanic episodes. Paradoxically, there have also been reports of hypomania on withdrawal of antidepressants, such as trazodone (Theilman and Christenbury, 1986) and desipramine (Nelson *et al*, 1983).

There have also been reports of mania induced by other psychiatric drugs, such as buspirone (McIvor and Sinanan, 1991) and risperidone (Schnierow and Graeber, 1996).

Other drugs used in general medicine (or otherwise) that have been implicated in the production of a hypomanic episode include: nasal decongestants (Wood, 1994); fenfluramine and phentermine (Raison and Klein, 1997); beclomethasone (Phelan, 1989) and anabolic-androgenic steroids (Pope and Katz, 1994); gabapentin (Hauck and Bhaumik, 1995), although gabapentin has also been used in the treatment of mania (Schaffer and Schaffer, 1997; Stanton *et al*, 1997); captopril (Gajula and Berlin, 1993); chloroquine (Lovestone, 1991); gonadotropin induction of ovulation (Persaud and Lam, 1998); and withdrawal of propranolol (Jouvent *et al*, 1986) and interferon-alfa (Carpiniello *et al*, 1998).

Social circumstances

Patients with both unipolar and bipolar disorder show decline in income and job status and all other areas of psychosocial functioning in the five years following an index episode. Even those who had a two-year period without symptoms did not report an improvement in income and job status. (Coryell *et al*, 1993).

Mental state examination

Patients with bipolar affective disorder tend to have suicidal feelings when there are strong depressive symptoms, either in the depressive swing or when a predominantly manic presentation is mixed with depressive features. Very occasionally, a patient with a manic state has suicidal ideation (Dilsaver *et al*, 1994). This is borne out by a study of completed suicides, in which the majority of patients with bipolar disorder (79%) committed suicide while in a depressive episode, 11% in a mixed state and 11% during or immediately following remission from psychotic mania (Isometsa *et al*, 1994).

There is evidence that the cognitive deficits notable in schizophrenia on measures of attention and psychomotor speed, verbal and visual memory and problem solving and abstraction are not present in affective disorder. IQ is lower in the schizophrenic group and appeared to have deteriorated from a normal pre-morbid level, unlike patients with affective disorder. However, patients with active symptoms of affective disorder show impaired performance on neuro- psychological testing (Goldberg *et al*, 1993). Van Gorp *et al*, (1998) found some evidence of impairment of verbal memory in bipolar patients, even when euthymic, but evidence of frontal-lobe executive dysfunction only in those patients with a history of alcohol dependence. The presence of clinical evidence of cognitive impairment in patients with bipolar disorder is associated with a pattern of subcortical brain morphologic abnormalities on magnetic resonance imaging (Dupont *et al*, 1995). There is evidence that reading and spelling ability are maintained even when IQ is lowered in schizophrenia and mania, giving a useful indication of pre-morbid intelligence (Dalby and Williams, 1986).

Management

Medication

Patients with bipolar affective disorder have elevations of D2 dopamine receptor Bmax values. Such elevations in affective disorder are more closely associated with the presence of psychosis than with mood abnormality (Pearlson *et al*, 1995). There is also clinical evidence that neuroleptics treat psychosis and lithium treats mood symptoms in a distinct manner (Johnstone *et al*, 1988). This provides a scientific rationale for the use of neuroleptics, such as haloperidol in the treatment of the acutely psychotic patient whose primary diagnosis is of an affective disorder. There is evidence that a dose of 10mg haloperidol daily is sufficient to treat patients with acute mania who will respond and that higher daily doses are ineffective (Rifkin *et al*, 1994). As such, there is some evidence that depot neuroleptics may be of value in the prophylactic treatment of patients with bipolar affective disorder (Littlejohn *et al*, 1994).

Evidence suggests that lithium is marginally better than carbamazepine in the treatment of acute mania, whereas carbamazepine is better prophylactically (Luznat *et al*, 1988). Sodium valproate has been used as monotherapy in acute mania. Bowden *et al* (1996) suggested that a serum level between 45 and 100–125mg/ml was associated with greater anti-manic efficacy with acceptable levels of side-effects. There is some suggestion that patients who have a depressive component to an acute manic episode respond better to sodium valproate than to lithium (Swann *et al*, 1997). Patients might be expected to respond within one in four days of achieving adequate valproate levels (Pope *et al*, 1991).

There have been case reports suggesting that clonidine may be useful in the treatment of acute mania (Maguire and Singh, 1987); there have also been reports of the use of lamotrigine (Labbate and Rubey, 1997; Kusumakar and Yatham, 1997) and clozapine (Calabrese *et al*, 1996) in treatment of refractory patients. For patients who do not respond to one drug, mood-stabilising drugs are often combined. Such combinations can be useful, but have potential dangers. There is some evidence of efficacy of combination of lithium with anticonvulsants, especially sodium valproate (Freeman and Stoll, 1998). For some particularly refractory patients, there may even be some benefit from triple therapy of lithium, carbamazepine and sodium valproate (Denicoff *et al*, 1997). A discussion of prophylaxis with lithium and other drugs can be found under the section on Depression.

A history of a being less accepting of medication for bipolar disorder is associated with an increased risk of readmission after the index episode (Joyce, 1985).

ECT

ECT has been tried in the treatment of mania. A review of the use of ECT in mania suggested that response could be obtained in 80% of patients in an episode of acute mania that had not responded to pharmacotherapy (Mukherjee *et al*, 1994). Following recovery from an acute episode, the use of maintenance ECT has been tried (Husain *et al*, 1993). There is also some evidence for a therapeutic advantage in the combination of chlorpromazine and ECT in the treatment of mania (Sidkar *et al*, 1994).

Psychosurgery

There is some experience of the use of psychosurgery in treatment resistant mania (Lovett and Shaw, 1987; Poynton *et al*, 1988; Sachdev *et al*, 1988).

Psychotherapy

Scott (1995) notes the limitations of pharmacotherapy in the treatment of hypomania and points out that there may be a number of psychological factors, consideration and treatment of which may improve outcome. These are in problems arising from the disorder, such as adjustment problems; loss (financial, employment, hope for the future, etc) and interpersonal relations, and in problems relating to compliance with medication. She pointed out that there may be some benefit from cognitive therapy, couple and group therapy and family therapy in the form of psychoeducation. She noted that the studies in relation to this area are unsophisticated and small.

References

Altshuler LL, Post RM, Leverich GS, Mikalauskas K, Rosoff A, Ackerman L (1995) Antidepressant-induced mania and cycle acceleration: a controversy revisited. *Am J Psychiatry* 152: 1130–8

Bamrah JS, Johnson J (1991) Bipolar affective disorder following head injury. *Br J Psychiatry* **158**: 117–9

Barczak P, Edmunds E, Betts T (1988) Hypomania following complex partial seizures. A report of three cases. *Br J Psychiatry* **152**: 137–9

Bauer MS, Whybrow PC, Winokur A (1990) Rapid cycling bipolar affective disorder. I. Association with grade I hypothyroidism. *Arch Gen Psychiatry* **47**: 427–32

Bell CC, Thompson B, Shakoor B (1987) Mania and head trauma. *Am J Psychiatry* **144**: 1378–9

Bellivier F, Leboyer M, Courtet P *et al* (1998) A. Association between the tryptophan hydroxylase gene and manic-depressive illness. *Arch Gen Psychiatry* **55**: 33–7

Benazzi F (1991) Uraemia and mania. *Br J Psychiatry* **158**: 718

Berrettini WH, Goldin LR, Gelernter J, Gejman PV, Gershon ES, Detera-Wadleigh S (1990) X-chromosome markers and manic-depressive illness. Rejection of linkage to Xq28 in nine bipolar pedigrees. *Arch Gen Psychiatry* **47**: 366–73

Berrettini WH, Ferraro TN, Goldin LR *et al* (1997) A linkage study of bipolar illness. *Arch Gen Psychiatry* **54**: 27–35

Berthier ML (1992) Post-stroke rapid cycling bipolar affective disorder. *Br J Psychiatry* **160**: 283

Berthier ML, Kulisevsky J (1993) Fluoxetine-induced mania in a patient with post-stroke depression. *Br J Psychiatry* **163**: 698–9

Blackwell MJ (1991) Rapid-cycling manic-depressive illness following subarachnoid haemorrhage. *Br J Psychiatry* **159**:279–80

Bowden CL, Janicak PG, Orsulak P *et al* (1996) Relation of serum valproate concentration to response in mania. *Am J Psychiatry* **153**: 765–70

Bracken P (1987) Mania following head injury. *Br J Psychiatry* **150**: 690–2

Brouillette MJ, Chouinard G, Lalonde R (1994) Didanosine-induced mania in HIV infection. *Am J Psychiatry* **151**: 1839–40

Bryois C, Ferrero F (1994) Mania induced by citalopram. *Arch Gen Psychiatry* **51**: 664–5

Buckley P, Hutchinson M (1993) Psychosis and multiple sclerosis. *Br J Psychiatry* **162**: 422–3

Byrne A (1988) Hypomania following increased epileptic activity. *Br J Psychiatry* **153**: 573–4

Calabrese JR, Kimmel SE, Woyshville MJ *et al* (1996) Clozapine for treatment-refractory mania. *Am J Psychiatry* **153**: 759–64

Calache MJ, Bourgeois M (1990) Bipolar affective disorder and anoxic brain damage. *Br J Psychiatry* **157**: 458–9

Cannon M, Jones P, Gilvarry C *et al* (1997) pre-morbid social functioning in schizophrenia and bipolar disorder: similarities and differences. *Am J Psychiatry* **154**: 1544–50

Carney PA, Fitzgerald CT, Monaghan CE (1988) Influence of climate on the prevalence of mania. *Br J Psychiatry* **152**: 820–23

Carpiniello B, Orru MG, Baita A, Pariante CM, Farci G (1998) Mania induced by withdrawal of treatment with interferon alfa. *Arch Gen Psychiatry* **55**: 88–9

Cassidy F, Forest K, Murray E, Carroll BJ (1998) A factor analysis of the signs and symptoms of mania. *Arch Gen Psychiatry* **55**: 27–32

Chawla M, Lindesay J (1993) Polycythaemia, delirium and mania. *Br J Psychiatry* **162**: 833–5

Chen YW, Dilsaver SC (1995) Comorbidity of panic disorder in bipolar illness: evidence from the Epidemiologic Catchment Area Survey. *Am J Psychiatry* **152**: 280–2

Christensen RC (1995) psychotic mania. *Am J Psychiatry* **152**: 1399–400

Chung RK, Langeluddecke P, Tennant C (1986) Threatening life events in the onset of schizophrenia, schizophreniform psychosis and hypomania. *Br J Psychiatry* **148**: 680–5

Clark AF, Davison K (1987) Mania following head injury. A report of two cases and a review of the literature. *Br J Psychiatry* **150**: 841–4

Collins MN, Jacobson RR (1990) Changing interactions between bipolar affective disorder and anoxic brain damage. *Br J Psychiatry* **156**: 736–40

Coryell W, Scheftner W, Keller M, Endicott J, Maser J, Klerman GL (1993) The enduring psychosocial consequences of mania and depression. *Am J Psychiatry* **150**: 720–7

Craddock N, Owen M (1992) Christmas disease and major affective disorder. *Br J Psychiatry* **160**: 715

Cummings JL, Mendez MF (1984) Secondary mania with focal cerebrovascular lesions. *Am J Psychiatry* **141**: 1084–7

Dalby JT, Williams R (1986) Preserved reading and spelling ability in psychotic disorders. *Psychol Med* **16**: 171–5

Dauncey K (1988) Mania in the early stages of AIDS. *Br J Psychiatry* **152**: 716–7

De Bruyn A, Mendelbaum K, Sandkuijl LA *et al* (1994) Nonlinkage of bipolar illness to tyrosine hydroxylase, tyrosinase, and D2 and D4 dopamine receptor genes on chromosome 11. *Am J Psychiatry* **151**: 102–6

Denicoff KD, Smith-Jackson EE, Bryan AL, Ali SO, Post RM (1997) Valproate prophylaxis in a prospective clinical trial of refractory bipolar disorder. *Am J Psychiatry* **154**: 1456–8

Dilsaver SC, Chen YW, Swann AC, Shoaib AM, Krajewski KJ (1994) Suicidality in patients with pure and depressive mania. *Am J Psychiatry* **151**: 1312–5

Dubin H, Spier S, Giannandrea P (1997) Nefazodone-induced mania. *Am J Psychiatry* **154**: 578–9

Dupont RM, Jernigan TL, Heindel W *et al* (1995) Magnetic resonance imaging and mood disorders. Localization of white matter and other subcortical abnormalities. *Arch Gen Psychiatry* **52**: 747–55

el-Badramany MH, Farag TI, al-Awadi SA, Hammad IM, Abdelkader A, Murthy DS (1989) Familial manic-depressive illness with deleted short arm of chromosome 21: coincidental or causal? *Br J Psychiatry* **155**: 856–7

Faedda GL, Tondo L, Teicher MH, Baldessarini RJ, Gelbard HA, Floris GF (1993) Seasonal mood disorders. Patterns of seasonal recurrence in mania and depression. *Arch Gen Psychiatry* **50**: 17–23

Freeman MP, Stoll AL (1998 Mood stabilizer combinations: a review of safety and efficacy. *Am J Psychiatry* **155**: 12–21

Gajula RP, Berlin RM (1993) Captopril-induced mania. *Am J Psychiatry* **150**: 1429–30

Gill M, Castle D, Duggan C (1992) Cosegregation of Christmas disease and major affective disorder in a pedigree. *Br J Psychiatry* **160**: 112–4

Goff DC (1985) Two cases of hypomania following the addition of L-tryptophan to a monoamine oxidase inhibitor. *Am J Psychiatry* **142**: 1487–8

Goggans FC (1984) A case of mania secondary to vitamin B12 deficiency. *Am J Psychiatry* **141**: 300–1

Goldberg TE, Gold JM, Greenberg R *et al* (1993) Contrasts between patients with affective disorders and patients with schizophrenia on a neuropsychological test battery. *Am J Psychiatry 150*: 1355–62

Gutierrez B, Bertranpetit J, Guillamat R *et al* (1997) Association analysis of the catechol O-methyltransferase gene and bipolar affective disorder. *Am J Psychiatry* **154**: 113–5

Hammen C, Gitlin M (1997) Stress reactivity in bipolar patients and its relation to prior history of disorder. *Am J Psychiatry* **154**: 856–7

Harrison-Read PE (1998) Lithium withdrawal mania supports lithium's action and suggests an animal model involving serotonin. *Br J Psychiatry* **172**: 96–7

Harvey NS, Mikhail WI (1986) Seasonal hypomania in a patient with cold urticaria. *Br J Psychiatry* **149**: 238–41

Haskett therefore (1985) Diagnostic categorization of psychiatric disturbance in Cushing's syndrome. *Am J Psychiatry* **142**: 911–6

Hauck A, Bhaumik S (1995) Hypomania induced by gabapentin. *Br J Psychiatry* **167**: 549

Haywood TW, Kravitz HM, Grossman LS, Cavanaugh JL Jr, Davis JM, Lewis DA (1995) Predicting the 'revolving door' phenomenon among patients with schizophrenic, schizoaffective, and affective disorders. *Am J Psychiatry* **152**: 856–61

Hebebrand J (1992) A critical appraisal of X-linked bipolar illness. Evidence for the assumed mode of inheritance is lacking. *Br J Psychiatry* **160**: 7–11

Holmes D, Brynjolfsson J, Brett P *et al* (1991) No evidence for a susceptibility locus predisposing to manic depression in the region of the dopamine (D2) receptor gene. *Br J Psychiatry* **158**: 635–41

Howland RH (1993) Bipolar disorder associated with primary generalised epilepsy. *Br J Psychiatry* **162**: 699–700

Husain MM, Meyer DE, Muttakin MH, Weiner MF (1993) Maintenance ECT for treatment of recurrent mania. *Am J Psychiatry* **150**: 985

Isles LJ, Orrell MW (1991) Secondary mania after open-heart surgery. *Br J Psychiatry* **159**: 280–82

Isometsa ET, Henriksson MM, Aro HM, Lonnqvist JK (1994) Suicide in bipolar disorder in Finland. *Am J Psychiatry* **151**: 1020–4

Jabeen S, Fisher CJ (1991) Trazodone-induced transient hypomanic symptoms and their management. *Br J Psychiatry* **158**: 275–8

Jampala VC, Abrams R (1983) Mania secondary to left and right hemisphere damage. *Am J Psychiatry* **140**: 1197–9

Johnson BA, Campbell LB (1990) Mood disorder, 'pre-ictal' psychosis and temporal lobe damage. *Br J Psychiatry* **157**: 441–4

Johnstone EC, Crow TJ, Frith CD, Owens DGC (1988) The Northwick Park 'functional' psychosis study: diagnosis and treatment response. *Lancet* ii: 119–25

Jorge RE, Robinson , Starkstein SE, Arndt SV, Forrester AW, Geisler FH (1993) Secondary mania following traumatic brain injury. *Am J Psychiatry* **150**: 916–21

Jouvent R, Baruch P, Simon P (1986) Manic episode after propranolol withdrawal. *Am J Psychiatry* **143**: 1633

Joyce PR (1985) Illness behaviour and in bipolar affective disorder. *Psychol Med* **15**: 521–5

Keck PE Jr, McElroy SL, Strakowski SM *et al* (1998) 12-month outcome of patients with bipolar disorder following hospitalization for a manic or mixed episode. *Am J Psychiatry* **155**: 646–52

Kendler KS, Pedersen N, Johnson L, Neale MC, Mathe AA (1993) A pilot Swedish twin study of affective illness, including hospital- and population-ascertained subsamples. *Arch Gen Psychiatry* **50**: 699–700

Kessing LV, Andersen PK, Mortensen PB, Bolwig TG (1998) Recurrence in affective disorder. I. Case register study. *Br J Psychiatry* **172**: 23–8

Kumar A, Agarwal M (1988) Secondary affective disorder in survivor of cardiac arrest. A case report. *Br J Psychiatry* **153**: 836–9

Kupfer DJ, Carpenter LL, Frank E (1988) Possible role of antidepressants in precipitating mania and hypomania in recurrent depression. *Am J Psychiatry* **145**: 804–8

Kusumakar V, Yatham LN (1997) Lamotrigine treatment of rapid cycling bipolar disorder. *Am J Psychiatry* **154**: 1171–2

Labbate LA, Rubey RN (1997) Lamotrigine for treatment-refractory bipolar disorder. *Am J Psychiatry* **154**: 1317

Laporta M, Chouinard G, Goldbloom D, Beauclair L (1987) Hypomania induced by sertraline, a new serotonin reuptake inhibitor. *Am J Psychiatry* **144**: 1513–4

Lee S, Chow CC, Wing YK, Leung CM, Chiu H, Chen CN (1991) Mania secondary to thyrotoxicosis. *Br J Psychiatry* **159**: 712–3

Littlejohn R, Leslie F, Cookson J (1994) Depot antipsychotics in the prophylaxis of bipolar affective disorder. *Br J Psychiatry* **165**: 827–9

Lovestone S (1991) Chloroquine-induced mania. *Br J Psychiatry* **159**: 164–5

Lovett LM, Shaw DM (1987) Outcome in bipolar affective disorder after tractotomy. *Br J Psychiatry* **151**: 113–6

Lusznat RM, Murphy DP, Nunn CM (1988) Carbamazepine vs lithium in the treatment and prophylaxis of mania. *Br J Psychiatry* **153**: 198–204

Lyketsos CG, Hanson AL, Fishman M, Rosenblatt A, McHugh PR, Treisman GJ (1993) Manic syndrome early and late in the course of HIV. *Am J Psychiatry* **150**: 326–7

Maguire J, Singh AN (1987) Clonidine. An effective anti-manic agent? *Br J Psychiatry* **150**: 863–4

McGuffin P, Katz R (1989) The genetics of depression and manic-depressive disorder. *Br J Psychiatry* **155**: 294–304

McIvor R, Sinanan K (1991) Buspirone-induced mania. *Br J Psychiatry* **158**: 136–7

McKeown SP, Jani CJ (1987) Mania following head injury. *Br J Psychiatry* **151**: 867–8

McLoughlin D, McKeon P (1991) Bipolar disorder and cerebral sarcoidosis. *Br J Psychiatry* **158**: 410–3

McPherson H, Herbison P, Romans S (1993) Life events and relapse in established bipolar affective disorder. *Br J Psychiatry* **163**: 381–5

Mendlewicz J (1992) X-linked bipolar illness. *Br J Psychiatry* **161**: 569–70

Mukherjee S, Sackeim HA, Schnur DB (1994) Electroconvulsive therapy of acute manic episodes: a review of 50 years' experience. *Am J Psychiatry* **151**: 169–76

Nelson JC, Schottenfeld RS, Conrad CD (1983) Hypomania after desipramine withdrawal. *Am J Psychiatry* **140**: 624–5

O'Connell RA, Mayo JA, Flatow L, Cuthbertson B, O'Brien BE (1991) Outcome of bipolar disorder on long-term treatment with lithium. *Br J Psychiatry* **159**: 123–9

Papolos DF, Faedda GL, Veit S *et al* (1996) Bipolar spectrum disorders in patients diagnosed with velo-cardio-facial syndrome: does a hemizygous deletion of chromosome 22q11 result in bipolar affective disorder? *Am J Psychiatry* **153**: 1541–7

Pearlson GD, Wong DF, Tune LE *et al* (1995) In vivo D2 dopamine receptor density in psychotic and nonpsychotic patients with bipolar disorder. *Arch Gen Psychiatry* **52**: 471–7

Persaud RN, Lam RW (1998) Manic reaction after induction of ovulation with gonadotropins. *Am J Psychiatry* **155**: 447–8

Peselow ED, Sanfilipo MP, Fieve RR (1995) Relationship between hypomania and personality disorders before and after successful treatment. *Am J Psychiatry* **152**: 232–8

Phelan MC (1989) Beclomethasone mania. *Br J Psychiatry* **155**: 871–2

Pickar D, Murphy DL, Cohen RM, Campbell IC, Lipper S (1982) Selective and nonselective monoamine oxidase inhibitors: behavioral disturbances during their administration to depressed patients. *Arch Gen Psychiatry* **39**: 535–40

Pope HG Jr, SL, Keck PE Jr, Hudson JI (1991) Valproate in the treatment of acute mania. A placebo-controlled study. *Arch Gen Psychiatry* **48**: 62–8

Pope HG Jr, Katz D (1994) Psychiatric and medical effects of anabolic-androgenic steroid use. A controlled study of 160 athletes. *Arch Gen Psychiatry* **51**: 375–82

Poynton A, Bridges PK, Bartlett JR (1988) Resistant bipolar affective disorder treated by stereotactic subcaudate tractotomy. *Br J Psychiatry* **152**: 354–8

Raison CL, Klein HM (1997) Psychotic mania associated with and phentermine use. *Am J Psychiatry* **154**: 711

Ram A, Guedj F, Cravchik A *et al* (1997) No abnormality in the gene for the G protein stimulatory alpha subunit in patients with bipolar disorder. *Arch Gen Psychiatry* **54**: 44–8

Rifkin A, Doddi S, Karajgi B, Borenstein M, Munne R (1994) Dosage of haloperidol for mania. *Br J Psychiatry* **165**: 113–6

Robinson RG, Boston JD, Starkstein SE, Price TR (1988) Comparison of mania and depression after brain injury: causal factors. *Am J Psychiatry* **145**: 172–8

Sachdev P, Smith JS, Matheson J (1988) Psychosurgery for bipolar affective disorder. *Br J Psychiatry* **153**: 576

Sanders RD, Deshpande AS (1990) Mania complicating ECT. *Br J Psychiatry* **157**: 153–4

Sax KW, Strakowski SM, Keck PE Jr *et al* (1997) Comparison of patients with early-, typical-, and late-onset affective psychosis. *Am J Psychiatry* **154**: 1299–301

Schaffer CB, Schaffer LC (1997) Gabapentin in the treatment of bipolar disorder. *Am J Psychiatry* **154**: 291–2

Schmidt U, Miller D (1988) Two cases of hypomania in AIDS. *Br J Psychiatry* **152**: 839–42

Schneider U, Malmadier A, Dengler R, Sollmann WP, Emrich HM (1996) Mood cycles associated with normal pressure hydrocephalus. *Am J Psychiatry* **153**: 1366–7

Schnierow BJ, Graeber DA (1996) Manic symptoms associated with initiation of risperidone. *Am J Psychiatry* **153**: 1235–6

Sclare P, Creed F (1990) Life events and the onset of mania. *Br J Psychiatry* **156**: 508–14

Scott J (1995) Psychotherapy for bipolar disorder. *Br J Psychiatry* **167**: 581–8

Scull DA, Trimble MR (1995) Mania precipitated by carbamazepine withdrawal. *Br J Psychiatry* **167**: 698

Shukla S, Cook BL, Mukherjee S, Godwin C, Miller MG (1987) Mania following head trauma. *Am J Psychiatry* **144**: 93–6

Sikdar S, Kulhara P, Avasthi A, Singh H (1994) Combined chlorpromazine and electroconvulsive therapy in mania. *Br J Psychiatry* **164**: 806–10

Singh AN, Maguire J (1988) Bipolar affective disorder and thalassemia minor — a genetic linkage? *Br J Psychiatry* **152**: 581

Smyth C, Kalsi G, Brynjolfsson J *et al* (1996) Further tests for linkage of bipolar affective disorder to the tyrosine hydroxylase gene locus on chromosome 11p15 in a new series of multiplex British affective disorder pedigrees. *Am J Psychiatry* **153**: 271–4

Snowdon J (1991) A retrospective case-note study of bipolar disorder in old age. *Br J Psychiatry* **158**: 485–90

Stanton SP, Keck PE Jr, McElroy SL (1997) Treatment of acute mania with gabapentin. *Am J Psychiatry* **154**: 287

Starkstein SE, Robinson RG (1989) Affective disorders and cerebral vascular disease. *Br J Psychiatry* **154**: 170–82

Steiner W (1991) Fluoxetine-induced mania in a patient with obsessive-compulsive disorder. *Am J Psychiatry* **148**: 1403–4

Stoll AL, Mayer PV, Kolbrener M *et al* (1994) Antidepressant-associated mania: a controlled comparison with spontaneous mania. *Am J Psychiatry* **151**: 1642–5

Stone K (1989) Mania in the elderly. *Br J Psychiatry* **155**: 220–4

Strakowski SM, Keck PE Jr, McElroy SL *et al* (1998) Twelve-month outcome after a first hospitalization for affective psychosis. *Arch Gen Psychiatry* **55**: 49–55

Sturdy JL, Mahapatra SB (1988) Mianserin and mania. *Br J Psychiatry* **153**: 269–70

Swann AC, Bowden CL, Morris D *et al* (1997) Depression during mania. Treatment response to lithium or divalproex. *Arch Gen Psychiatry* **54**: 37–42

Theilman SB, Christenbury MM (1986) Hypomania following withdrawal of trazodone. *Am J Psychiatry* **143**: 1482–3

Thienhaus OJ, Khosla N (1984) Meningeal cryptococcosis misdiagnosed as a manic episode. *Am J Psychiatry* **141**: 1459–60

Thomas CS, Neale TJ (1991) Organic manic syndrome associated with advanced uraemia due to polycystic kidney disease. *Br J Psychiatry* **158**: 119–21

Tohen M, Shulman KI, Satlin A (1994) First-episode mania in late life. *Am J Psychiatry* **151**: 130–2

Turecki G, Mari J de J, Del Porto JA (1993) Bipolar disorder following a left basal-ganglia stroke. *Br J Psychiatry* **163**: 690

van Gorp WG, Altshuler L, Theberge DC, Wilkins J, Dixon W (1998) Cognitive impairment in euthymic bipolar patients with and without prior alcohol dependence. A preliminary study. *Arch Gen Psychiatry* **55**: 41–6

van Os J, Jones P, Lewis G, Wadsworth M, Murray R (1997) Developmental precursors of affective illness in a general population birth cohort. *Arch Gen Psychiatry* **54**: 625–31

Walbridge DG (1990) Rapid-cycling disorder in association with cerebral sarcoidosis. *Br J Psychiatry* **157**: 611–13

Winokur G, Coryell W, Akiskal HS *et al* (1995a) Alcoholism in manic-depressive (bipolar) illness: familial illness, course of illness, and the primary-secondary distinction. *Am J Psychiatry* **152**: 365–72

Winokur G, Coryell W, Keller M, Endicott J, Leon A (1995b) A family study of manic-depressive (bipolar I) disease. Is it a distinct illness separable from primary unipolar depression? *Arch Gen Psychiatry* **52**: 367–73

Wood KA (1994) Nasal decongestant and psychiatric disturbance. *Br J Psychiatry* **164**: 566–7

Wright JB (1993) Mania following sleep deprivation. *Br J Psychiatry* **163**: 679–80

Wylie K, de Silva D, Jerram T, Mindham RH (1993) Simultaneous kidney disease and manic-depressive psychosis. *Br J Psychiatry* **162**: 275–6

Yatham LN (1987) Mania following head injury. *Br J Psychiatry* **151**: 558

Yuvarajan R, Yousufzai NM (1988) Mania induced by lithium augmentation. A case report. *Br J Psychiatry* **153**: 828–30

Zmitek A (1987) Trazodone-induced mania. *Br J Psychiatry* **151**: 274–5

7

Mental handicap

Mental handicap (learning difficulties)

- ◆ An informant may be present

History of presenting complaint

The patient may already have been diagnosed by the paediatricians and been transferred to the care of psychiatrists with special interest in mental handicap at the age of 16 years. The patient may come to attention because of:

- ◆ Acute physical illness
- ◆ Behavioural disturbance
    - ❑ difficult or obstreperous behaviour
    - ❑ angry outburst
    - ❑ violence to property or to people
      smashing a window
      arson
    - ❑ inappropriate sexual behaviour
      exposure
      sexual harassment
      promiscuity
    - ❑ superimposition of mental illness
- ◆ Increasing difficulty in coping by the carer
    - ❑ patient growing up
      and therefore being bigger and heavier to lift, dress etc.
    - ❑ carer growing older
      reduction in physical strength and therefore less able to lift
      carer burnout (psychologically)
    - ❑ family crisis leading to decompensation of coping
      breadwinner losing his / her job
      serious illness or death in a family member
- ◆ Change in the environment
    - ❑ closure of mental hospitals
    - ❑ changes in benefit regulations

Family history

- Increased maternal age
- History of Down's Syndrome

Personal history

- Infection *in utero*
  - ❑ TORCH
- Perinatal events
  - ❑ traumatic delivery
    anoxia
    foetal distress
  - ❑ periventricular haemorrhage
  - ❑ epileptic fits
  - ❑ spontaneous hypoglycaemic attacks
  - ❑ hypothyroidism
  - ❑ phenylketonuria
- Delayed walking
- Delayed speech
- Loss of acquired skills
- Attendance at a special school
- History of irresponsible or unwise behaviour
- Failure to develop a work career or work in protected environments

Past medical history

- Infection, encephalitis, or meningitis as a child
- Severe head injury
  - ❑ road traffic accident
  - ❑ fall from a height
  - ❑ postoperative
  - ❑ non-accidental injury
- History of epilepsy
- History of congenital cardiac abnormalities and operation
- Illnesses associated with bony deformities
  - ❑ eg. recurrent chest infections

Past psychiatric history

- ◆ Concomitant psychiatric illness
  - ❑ schizophrenia
  - ❑ bipolar affective disorder
  - ❑ Alzheimer's disease

Drug history

- ◆ Long-term prophylactic antibiotics
- ◆ Anti-epileptic medication

Pre-morbid personality

- ◆ History of period of development as a normal child before damage occurring
  - ❑ autism
  - ❑ prior to major event leading to brain damage

Social circumstances

- ◆ Residence in a group home or hostel

Psychosexual history

- ◆ May not have had any sexual partners
- ◆ May have had a period of promiscuity followed by birth of a child given up for adoption

Mental state examination

Appearance

- ◆ Facial dysmorphism
- ◆ Physical concomitants of syndromes, for example:
  - ❑ simian crease
  - ❑ obesity
- ◆ Musculoskeletal abnormalities
  - ❑ crooked chest
  - ❑ abnormal hand or leg postures
  - ❑ patient sitting in a wheelchair

- Patient appears of low intelligence

Behaviour

- Repetitive movements
  - ❏ especially if autistic — great distress caused if interrupted
- Non-verbal communication
  - ❏ eg. greater use of pointing at things
- May show inappropriate social body language
  - ❏ eg. lack of fear of strangers

Mood

- Normal, in the absence of other suggestion of mental illness

Affect

- Smiling/warm
- Fatuous grin

Speech

- May be absent
- Nasal/dysarthric
- Speech may contain language suggestive of low intelligence

Thoughts and experiences

- Normal, in the absence of concomitant mental illness

Cognition

- Disorientation in time, but not always in place
- Many skills required for routine cognitive testing may be absent
  - ❏ inability to write
  - ❏ inability to calculate
  - ❏ lack of awareness of external events and limited general knowledge

Insight

- Not relevant

Investigations and management

- ◆ Diagnosis of syndrome
  - ❑ chromosomal analysis
    trisomy
    fragile X
- ◆ Assess disabilities
  - ❑ WAIS testing
  - ❑ assessment of activities of daily living
- ◆ Assess residual abilities
- ◆ Monitor and treat epilepsy
- ◆ Prophylactic antibiotics
- ◆ Support for patient
  - ❑ easy access to counselling
    practical life skills
    support against stigma
  - ❑ advice about budgeting
  - ❑ advice about practical issues
  - ❑ advice about sex
    contraception
    appropriate and inappropriate behaviours
- ■ Assessing suitable and willing partners
- ■ Assessing consent to sex
    dealing with the prejudices of others
- ◆ Residence
  - ❑ hospital
  - ❑ hostel
  - ❑ group home
  - ❑ with parents/family
  - ❑ independent living, with or without spouse/partner
- ◆ Occupation
  - ❑ independent employment
  - ❑ without support
  - ❑ with support from professionals preferably through the company doctor
  - ❑ sheltered work
  - ❑ day centres; social clubs
  - ❑ occupational therapy
- ◆ Finances
  - ❑ ensure all benefits to which the patient is entitled are claimed

- ☐ assist with budgeting
- ◆ Speech therapy
- ◆ Physiotherapy
  - ☐ chest
  - ☐ limbs for contractures
- ◆ Support for families/carers
  - ☐ information and education
  - ☐ counselling
  - ☐ respite care
- ◆ Self-help groups
  - ☐ SCOPE
  - ☐ MENCAP

✱   ✱   ✱   ✱   ✱

'A rose by any other name would smell as sweet.' Stigma is like roses. You can change the name, but people soon find out. Mental handicap or the fashionable term 'learning disabilities' — has gone through just such changes. 'Idiot' at the turn of the twentieth century; 'spastic'; 'educationally subnormal (ESN)'. These terms do not disguise a group that is consistently stigmatised. We need to change people's attitudes, not names.

Mental handicap (the term I will use throughout this section, even though it is politically incorrect) is a term used to indicate interruption in the development of the brain and higher structures of the central nervous system. In contrast, **dementia** is a loss of acquired mental function; **mental handicap** is the failure to develop the function in the first place.

Origins of mental handicap can be congenital or acquired. Certain chromosomal abnormalities, most notably trisomy 21 (Down's Syndrome), can cause mental handicap. So can infections in the womb (the TORCH infections — toxoplasmosis, rubella, cytomegalovirus and herpes zoster [chicken pox] — are the best known) or birth trauma, such as failure of oxygenation leading to periventricular haemorrhage. In childhood, an encephalitis or meningitis, or a severe head injury, caused in a road traffic accident or by beatings from a physically abusive parent, can arrest the development of a child that would otherwise have been normal.

The diagnosis may be made in the womb by amniocentesis (insertion of a needle into the womb to draw off a little amniotic fluid) and examination of cells found in the amniotic fluid. It may become obvious at birth, because of the unusual facial characteristics of the baby ('mongoloid features') in Down's syndrome. Down's syndrome is associated with many other abnormalities, most notably congenital cardiac abnormalities. After birth, a child that appears normal may develop epileptic fits or attacks of hypoglycaemia (low blood sugar). As the child matures, he/she may show evidence of retarded development: he or she might not walk at the right age; speech development may be very slow, limited to a few words or be non-existent. In childhood, this is sad, but tolerable; it becomes much harder for a parent to manage when the child reaches adulthood and may be unable to look after him/herself at all.

He/she could have difficulties dressing, feeding, urinating and defaecating, or may have limitations in some of these.

Not every person with mental handicap is unable to live independently. It is salutary to recall that a person with Down's syndrome has been known to obtain a university degree, although this is exceptional. Many people with mental handicap can live ordinary run-of-the-mill lives, appearing to others as dull, but otherwise relatively normal.

The speciality of mental handicap has established a professional body, with the expertise to help those who suffer from learning difficulties. Their knowledge ensures that treatment is offered that is appropriate to the needs of those with mild impairments, as well as to those who are severely disabled.

People with mental handicap need additional help obtaining necessities that others take for granted. Those with limited impairment may live independently and undertake manual tasks. However, carrying out complex social tasks, such as filling in forms or dealing with tax may be beyond their skills. Establishing interpersonal relationships may fail because of rigid thinking patterns and difficulty understanding aspects of living that require information and explanation, for example, aspects of sexuality. For these people, practical help budgeting their weekly income, filling in benefit forms and counselling is very helpful.

In contrast, those with almost complete absence of speech, epilepsy, or musculoskeletal abnormalities leading to inability to walk or move the limbs and thus inability to wash, dress or even feed themselves may need full-time nursing in residential accommodation.

Between these extremes are those who are able to look after their basic self-care and make informed choices about what they want, but are unable to cope in the outside world. They may require hostel accommodation with permanent residential staff, but limited supervision, or help in finding sheltered work or occupation in a day centre. They may have difficulty looking after their own financial and day-to-day affairs. In this group, a major problem is that a limited ability to speak and articulate complex thoughts limits communication to non-verbal methods. People inexperienced in dealing with those who suffer mental handicap can misinterpretate behaviour as mental illness when sufferers are only trying to communicate distress at their inability to verbalise their problems. Someone with learning disabilities has to rely on those around to understand what has happened. For example, if a person without a mental handicap were to have a piece of property taken away without explanation, the owner of the property might request the return of the property immediately. However, if a person with a mental handicap has his wallet removed without understanding that the care staff member was offering to put it in safe keeping, an understandable response might be to smash a window to indicate displeasure. Inexperienced carers immediately seek professional help, whereas a more experienced member of staff would realise what has happened, deal with the situation by offering an explanation to the client and an injunction not to smash things the next time the client is unhappy. Alternatively, the person with mental handicap who feels that he or she would like some company might do something socially unacceptable, like smashing a window, because he or she knows that this is usually followed by a response, giving him or her the attention he or she desires. Again, an experienced member of staff would recognise what had happened and take steps to prevent a recurrence, scolding the person for unacceptable behaviour, but looking for ways to meet the need for company in a more acceptable fashion.

Thus behaviour that might, in other patients, give rise to beliefs that he or she might be suffering from mental illness may have a more simple explanation in a patient with a mental handicap. However, it is becoming accepted that mental illness does occur in people with mental handicap in the same way as in those without mental handicap. In particular, it is felt that schizophrenia and bipolar affective disorder can arise in people with mental handicap, although diagnosis is more difficult because the patient usually cannot describe his or her symptoms. The diagnosis usually has to be made on external observations. In schizophrenia, there may be a noticeable deterioration in the personality. The person may becomes less responsive to others and less involved in self-care, interaction with others and motivation. Delusions and hallucinations can occur, but may be more simple than in those without mental handicap. Mood disorders may present with overactivity and giggling (suggesting hypomania) or underactivity, loss of appetite, constipation and the appearance of misery or unexplained crying (suggesting depression). Treatment for major mental illness is the same as that for those without a mental handicap, but there is a tendency to use pharmacological agents as dynamic psychotherapy is more difficult.

It is the role of the psychiatrist specialising in mental handicap to assess such situations, to decide whether there is a simple psychological explanation or a major mental disorder present, and to institute treatment accordingly.

✳   ✳   ✳   ✳   ✳

History of presenting complaint

Mental handicap may be a considered a discipline that is not the province of the psychiatrist. The diagnosis has often been made well before the patient reaches maturity. Some psychiatrists have tried to redefine the role by stating their expertise as the diagnosis and treatment of general adult psychiatric conditions (eg. schizophrenia, affective disorder) as they present in mental handicap. Although this is an important role of a psychiatrist in the management of patients with mental handicap, it is not the entire picture and other valuable contributions can be made. These include:

- diagnosis and treatment of general adult psychiatric conditions (eg. schizophrenia, affective disorder) as they present in mental handicap
- assessment of behavioural problems as they arise, clarifying the physical, medical, psychological and psychiatric contributions
- assessment and management of medical conditions common in this patient group, such as epilepsy or chest infections. A psychiatrist who knows a patient well may be in a better position to diagnose a chest infection than a physician who has not listened to the patient's chest before
- team leadership, integrating the social, psychological and physical care of the patient and the family. This is provided by diverse professionals, such as hospital and community nurses, occupational therapists, physiotherapists, speech therapists, psychologists and social workers

- acting as a resource for advice on specialist problems, such as the appropriate way an adult with mental handicap might gain a fulfilling sexual life and when ability to consent to intercourse might be compromised.

Thus, the doctor specialising in mental handicap is most likely to be involved when there is a crisis, although there is a role in the maintenance of stability by, for example, monitoring the control of epilepsy and ensuring arrangements are in place for provision of respite care. In the presentation of the patient to the psychiatrist, referral is most likely to occur because of a behavioural problem. The referral may arise in the community, or in a residential, hospital or forensic setting.

There are a range of behavioural disturbances (Reid and Ballinger, 1995), such as assault (Linaker, 1994), temper tantrums, unco-operativeness, attention-seeking, self-injury and property destruction, that occur frequently in a substantial minority (Smith *et al,* 1996). Behaviours, such as noisiness, social withdrawal and stripping can be persistent over many years (Reid and Ballinger, 1995). The specialist should be aware that such behaviours, while appearing random to a lay person, are often understandable, and precipitants of undesirable behaviour should be sought. For example, arguments with parents, bereavement, starting or ending a heterosexual relationship or leaving school and starting at a day centre may be followed by behavioural disturbance (Ghaziuddin, 1988). A person, whose development was not interrupted by a toxic process that caused brain damage, might express such distress in another form. It is also important to recognise that physical conditions, especially epilepsy, can present as behavioural disturbance (Deb and Hunter, 1991).

There are a number of behavioural difficulties that carers manage in the handicapped relatives they care for. However, it is behaviours where aggression is directed outward, such as aggression to self and others, disturbing noises, temper tantrums, etc, rather than passive behaviours, such as lethargy, stereotypy and inappropriate speech, that lead to referrals to specialist services (Lowe *et al*, 1995).

Family history

The genetic disorders that lead to mental handicap, such as Down's Syndrome, and the effects of increasing maternal age are well documented in medical and paediatric textbooks. A review can be found in Thapar *et al* (1994). Recently, interest has focussed on the Fragile X syndrome (Turk, 1992).

Autism seems to have a familial component, and there seems to be a mild phenotype in other members of the families of patients. Parents of patients with autism appear to be more aloof, tactless and unresponsive than the parents of controls (Piven *et al,* 1994). They also frequently exhibit more social and communication deficits and stereotyped behaviours (Piven *et al,* 1997).

Personal history

There may be evidence of failure of mental development in childhood by the time a patient reaches adulthood.

Past medical history

The physical illnesses associated with mental handicap are well documented in medical textbooks. They range from disorders that are associated with the condition, for example, hypothyroidism (Mani, 1988), to conditions that are secondary, such as chest infections as a result of abnormal development of the chest skeleton. Epilepsy is common among patients with a mental handicap and may require specialist management (McVicker *et al*, 1994; Deb and Hunter, 1991a-c).

Past psychiatric history

Detection of psychiatric disorder in mentally handicapped people can be difficult. See *Table 7.1* for a list of some psychiatric disorders. Reviews can be found in Linaker and Nitter (1990), Ballinger (1991), Collacott (1992) and Reid (1994).

Table 7.1: Psychiatric disorder in mental handicap	
Dementia	Moss and Patel, 1995
Manic-depressive illness	Arumainayagam and Kumar, 1990 Cook and Leventhal, 1987 Cooper and Collacott, 1993 McLaughlin, 1987
Depression	Ghaziuddin and Tsai, 1991 Jancar and Gunaratne, 1994
Suicidal behaviour	Walters, 1990
Disordered eating behaviour	O'Brien and Whitehouse, 1990
Pica	Jawed *et al*, 1993 McLoughlin, 1988
Eating disorders	Holt *et al*, 1988
OCD	McNally and Calamari, 1989
Personality disorder	Reid and Ballinger, 1987
Schizophrenia	Meadows *et al*, 1991

Historical analysis suggests the possibility that the incidence of psychotic illness is increased among people with intellectual retardation (Turner, 1989). With the increased longevity of people with mental handicap, evidence is appearing that older people with mental handicap have a higher incidence of mental illness than younger people. Older people show a higher incidence of anxiety disorders, depression and dementia, but equal rates for schizophrenia, delusional disorders, autism and behaviour disorders (Patel *et al*, 1993; Cooper, 1997).

The presentation of psychiatric disorder may be different in patients with mental handicap, who may make greater use of non-verbal means of expressing distress. In response to stress, patients may tend to show self-destructive or aggressive behaviour (Stack *et al*, 1987).

There is evidence that diagnosis of affective illness can be made according to DSM-III criteria in people with mental handicap (Sovner and Hurley, 1983), although Cooper and Collacott (1994) find the ICD-10 and DSM-IIIR criteria too restrictive. It would appear that psychogenic factors may precipitate mental disturbance: patients are not unaware of the stigma of mental handicap (Reiss and Benson, 1984). Furthermore, stresses such as physical or sexual abuse may precipitate psychoses (Varley, 1984; Martorana, 1985).

Pre-morbid personality

Forensic history

There is evidence that patients with mental handicap have a greater risk of committing criminal offences, especially violence, than the general population. (Hodgins, 1992). The risk factors for offending by people with learning disabilities appear to be the same as those in a non-mentally handicapped population (ie. family breakup, other family members with forensic contact, history of truancy and repeated offending) rather than arising out of mental handicap (Winter *et al*, 1997). There is also evidence of an over-representation of sex offences among the mentally handicapped, against a background of a high prevalence of family psychopathology, psychiatric illness, minor physical disabilities, sexual experience, impaired relationship skills and sexual recidivism (Day, 1994).

Mental state examination

Much observational information gathered in the clinical interaction with the patient will contribute to the diagnosis of mental handicap. In the examination for possible mental disorder, the clinician will need to consider behaviours rather than verbal accounts of experiences (eg. the presence of an hallucination may need to be inferred from behaviour rather than from the patient's account). Caution is needed to avoid over-interpreting the presence of abnormal experiences.

Management

Drugs — management of behavioural disturbance

It is never satisfactory to manage psychological distress by tranquillisation, but there are times when it is the least undesirable option. Neuroleptics have been used acutely (Malt *et al*, 1995) and so have benzodiazepines, such as midazolam (Bond *et al*, 1989). Lithium has been used in an attempt to reduce the seriousness of frequent aggressive outbursts (Craft *et al*, 1987), sometimes in combination with carbamazepine (Buck and Havey, 1986). More recently, overactivity of the endogenous opiate system has been postulated as a mechanism for self-injurious behaviour. There is some evidence of raised plasma and CSF endorphin levels (Gillberg *et al*, 1985; Willemsen-Swinkels *et al*, 1996) in patients with self-injurious behaviour, but a recent study testing this hypothesis failed to find a benefit for naltrexone in its treatment (Willemsen-Swinkels *et al*, 1995).

Psychological

Behavioural modification has long been used to assist mentally handicapped people whose behaviour presents difficulties. The family, including siblings, can be involved in behavioural modification (Miller and Cantwell, 1976). Social skills training may also be helpful (Brady, 1984).

Social — residential placement

There is evidence that moving patients out from long-stay hospitals to an NHS hostel in the community can lead to improvement in function. For less severely handicapped, more socially able patients, improvements in behaviour and activities of daily living were noted in one study on movement from a large hospital to a hostel. This was not found in the more severely handicapped who stayed behind (Shah and Holmes, 1987). This finding may be a product of the quality of the environment as much as the place. Assessment of discharged hospital residents with learning disabilities showed minimal change over two years when discharge has been predominantly to residential and nursing homes with a lack of 'ordinary' accommodation (Donnelly *et al*, 1996).

Needs of the family

The birth of a mentally handicapped child leads early psychological reactions in the family that can include a grief reaction and rejection of the child. Psychological difficulties do not cease in families who decide to keep the child, and some express this by a failure to let go of the child when he reaches adult age. Psychological and other family responses have been described (Davis, 1967; Fabrega and Haka, 1967; Blumenthal, 1969; Bicknell, 1983). Formal examination of how families cope in practice identifies five main coping strategies: practical coping; wishful thinking; stoicism; seeking emotional social support; passive acceptance (Knussen *et al*,1992). These strategies seem stable over time (Hatton *et al*, 1995).

The psychiatrist should be aware of these difficulties and of options both to support the family when they are coping, such as self-help groups, and when the family is decompensating, such as emergency respite care.

References

Arumainayagam M, Kumar A (1990) Manic-depressive psychosis in a mentally handicapped person. Seasonality: a clue to a diagnostic problem. *Br J Psychiatry* 156: 886

Ballinger BR, Ballinger CB, Reid AH, McQueen E (1991) The psychiatric symptoms, diagnoses and care needs of 100 mentally handicapped patients. *Br J Psychiatry* **158**: 251–4

Bicknell J (1983) The psychopathology of handicap. *Br J Med Psychol* **56**:167–78

Blumenthal MD (1969) Experiences of parents of retardates and children with cystic fibrosis. *Arch Gen Psychiatry* **21**: 160–71

Bond WS, Mandos LA, Kurtz MB (1989) Midazolam for aggressivity and violence in three mentally retarded patients. *Am J Psychiatry* **146**: 925–6

Brady JP (1984) Social skills training for psychiatric patients, II: Clinical outcome studies. *Am J Psychiatry* **141**: 491–8

Buck OD, Havey P (1986) Combined carbamazepine and lithium therapy for violent behavior. *Am J Psychiatry* **143**: 1487

Cook EH, Leventhal BL (1987) Down's syndrome with mania. *Br J Psychiatry* **150**: 249

Collacott RA, Cooper SA, McGrother C (1992) Differential rates of psychiatric disorders in adults with Down's Syndrome compared with other mentally handicapped adults. *Br J Psychiatry* **161**: 671–4

Cooper S-A, Collacott RA (1993) Mania and Down's syndrome. *Br J Psychiatry* **162**:739–43

Cooper SA, RA (1994) Clinical features and diagnostic criteria of depression in Down's syndrome. *Br J Psychiatry* **165**: 399–403

Cooper SA (1997) Epidemiology of psychiatric disorders in elderly compared with younger adults with learning disabilities. *Br J Psychiatry* **170**: 375–80

Craft M, Ismail IA, Krishnamurti D *et al*)1987) Lithium in the treatment of aggression in mentally handicapped patients. *Br J Psychiatry* **150**: 685–9

Davis DR (1967) Family processes in mental retardation. *Am J Psychiatry* **124**: 340–50

Day K (1994) Male mentally handicapped sex offenders. *Br J Psychiatry* **165**: 630–39

Deb S, Hunter D (1991a) Psychopathology of people with mental handicap and epilepsy. I: Maladaptive behaviour. *Br J Psychiatry* **159**: 822–6

Deb S, Hunter D (1991b) Psychopathology of people with mental handicap and epilepsy. II:Psychiatric illness. *Br J Psychiatry* **159**: 826–30

Deb S, Hunter D (1991c) Psychopathology of people with mental handicap and epilepsy. III: Personality disorder. *Br J Psychiatry* **159**: 830–34

Donnelly M, McGilloway S, Mays N *et al* (1996) One and two year outcomes for adults with learning disabilities discharged to the community. *Br J Psychiatry* **168**: 598–606

Fabrega H Jr, Haka KK (1967) Parents of mentally handicapped children. A social psychiatric case study. *Arch Gen Psychiatry* **16**: 202–9

Ghaziuddin M (1988) Behaviour disorder in the mentally handicapped: the role of life events. *Br J Psychiatry* **152**: 683–6

Ghaziuddin M, Tsai L (1991) Depression in autistic disorder. *Br J Psychiatry* **159**: 721

Gillberg C, Terenius L, Lonnerholm G (1985) Endorphin activity in childhood psychosis. Spinal fluid levels in 24 cases. *Arch Gen Psychiatry* **42**: 780–3

Hatton C, Knussen C, Sloper P, Turner S (1995) The stability of the Ways of Coping (Revised) Questionnaire over time in parents of children with Down's syndrome: a research note. *Psychol Med* **25**: 419–22

Hodgings S (1992) Mental disorder, intellectual deficiency, and crime. Evidence from a birth cohort. *Arch Gen Psychiatry* **49**: 476–83

Holt GM, N, Watson JP (1988) Down's syndrome and eating disorders: a case study. *Br J Psychiatry* **152**: 847

Jancar J, Gunaratne IJ (1994) Dysthymia and mental handicap. *Br J Psychiatry* **164**: 691

Jawed SH, Krishnan VHR, Prasher VP, Corbett JA (1993) Worsening of pica as a symptom of depressive illness in a person with severe mental handicap. *Br J Psychiatry* **162**: 835

Knussen C, Sloper P, Cunningham CC, Turner S (1992) The use of the Ways of Coping (Revised) questionnaire with parents of children with Down's syndrome. *Psychol Med* **22**: 775–86

Linaker OM, Nitter R (1990) Psychopathology in institutionalised mentally retarded adults. *Br J Psychiatry* **156**: 522–5

Linaker OM (1994) Assaultiveness among institutionalised adults with mental retardation. *Br J Psychiatry* **164**: 62–8

Lowe K, Felce D, Blackman D (1995) People with learning disabilities and challenging behaviour: the characteristics of those referred and not referred to specialist teams. *Psychol Med* **25**: 595–603

Malt UF, Nystad R, *et al* (1995) The effectiveness of zuclopenthixol compared with that of haloperidol in the treatment of behavioural disturbances in mentally retarded patients. A double-blind crossover study. *Br J Psychiatry* **166**: 374–7

Mani C (1988) Hypothyroidism in Down's syndrome. *Br J Psychiatry* **153**: 102

Martorana GR (1985) Schizophreniform disorder in a mentally retarded adolescent boy following sexual victimization. *Am J Psychiatry* **142**: 784

McLaughlin M (1987) Bipolar affective disorder in Down's syndrome *Br J Psychiatry* **151**: 116

McLoughlin IJ (1988) Pica as a cause of death in three mentally handicapped men. *Br J Psychiatry* **152**: 842

McNally RJ, Calamari JE (1989) Obsessive-compulsive disorder in a mentally retarded woman. *Br J Psychiatry* **155**: 116

McVicker RW, Shanks OEP, McLelland RJ (1994) Prevalence and associated features of epilepsy in adults with Down' syndrome. *Br J Psychiatry* **164**: 528–32

Meadows G, Turner T, Campbell L, Lewis SW, Reveley MA, Murray RM (1991) Assessing schizophrenia in adults with mental retardation. A comparative study. *Br J Psychiatry* **158**: 103

Miller NB, Cantwell DP (1976) Siblings as therapists: a behavioral approach. *Am J Psychiatry* **133**: 447–50

Moss S, Patel P (1995) Psychiatric symptoms associated with dementia in older people with learning disability. *Br J Psychiatry* **167**: 663

O'Brien G, Whitehouse AM (1990) A psychiatric study of deviant eating behaviour among mentally handicapped adults. *Br J Psychiatry* **157**: 281

Patel P, Goldberg D, Moss S (1993) Psychiatric morbidity in older people with moderate and severe learning disability. II: The prevalence study. *Br J Psychiatry* **163**: 481–91

Piven J, Wzorek M, Landa R *et al* (1994) Personality characteristics of the parents of autistic individuals. *Psychol Med* **24**: 783–95

Piven J, Palmer P, Jacobi D, Childress D, Arndt S (1997) Broader autism phenotype: evidence from a family history study of multiple-incidence autism families. *Am J Psychiatry* **154**: 185–90

Reid AH, Ballinger BR (1987) Personality disorder in mental handicap. *Psychol Med* **17**: 983–7

Reid AH (1994) Psychiatry and learning disability. *Br J Psychiatry* **164**: 613–8

Reid A, Ballinger BR (1995) Behaviour symptoms among severely and profoundly mentally retarded patients. A 16-18 year follow-up study. *Br J Psychiatry* **167**: 452–5

Reiss S, Benson BA (1984) Awareness of negative social conditions among mentally retarded, emotionally disturbed outpatients. *Am J Psychiatry* **141**: 88–90

Shah A, Holmes N (1987) Locally-based residential services for mentally handicapped adults: a comparative study. *Psychol Med* **17**: 763–74

Sovner R, Hurley AD (1983) Do the mentally retarded suffer from affective illness? *Arch Gen Psychiatry* **40**: 61–7

Stack LS, Haldipur CV, Thompson M (1987) Stressful life events and psychiatric hospitalization of mentally retarded patients. *Am J Psychiatry* **144**: 661–3

Thapar A, Gottesman II, Owen MJ, O'Donovan MC, McGuffin P (1994) The genetics of mental retardation. *Br J Psychiatry* **164**: 747–58

Turk J (1992) The fragile-X syndrome. On the way to a behavioural phenotype. *Br J Psychiatry* **160**: 24–35

Turner TH (1989) Schizophrenia and mental handicap: an historical review, with implications for further research. *Psychol Med* **19**: 301–14

Varley CK (1984) Schizophreniform psychoses in mentally retarded adolescent girls following sexual assault. *Am J Psychiatry* **141**: 593–5

Walters RM (1990) Suicidal behaviour in severely mentally handicapped patients. *Br J Psychiatry* **157**: 444

Willemsen-Swinkels SH, Buitelaar JK, Nijhof GJ, van England H (1995) Failure of naltrexone hydrochloride to reduce self-injurious and autistic behavior in mentally retarded adults. Double-blind placebo-controlled studies. *Arch Gen Psychiatry* **52**: 766–73

Willemsen-Swinkels SH, Buitelaar JK, Weijnen FG, Thijssen JH, Van Engeland H (1996) Plasma beta-endorphin concentrations in people with learning disability and self-injurious and/or autistic behaviour. *Br J Psychiatry* **168**: 105–9

Winter N, Holland AJ, Collins S (1997) Factors predisposing to suspected offending by adults with self-reported learning disabilities. *Psychol Med* **27**: 595–607

8

Obsessive-compulsive disorder

History

Obsessive-compulsive symptoms

◆ Obsession
  ❐ a senseless or repugnant intrusive or recurrent thought, image or impulse that the person attempts to ignore or suppress (Zetin and Kramer) and recognises as coming from within (PSE)

  obsessive thought; obsessive idea; obsessive rumination: eg. safety; knives; obscenities; ruminating on the meaning of the universe, fear of contamination or germs; fear of causing harm to self or others; fear of loss of control; pervasive doubts; sexual or religious fears
  obsessive slowness: secondary to rituals in the morning preparation, leaving one place for another, travelling rituals
  obsessive doubt

◆ Compulsion
  ❐ a need to perform a task or ritual in a repetitive, seemingly purposeful, stereotyped manner that is designed to produce or prevent some future event or situation. The act is not realistically connected to the event or situation and is usually viewed by the patient as excessive, senseless and unpleasant despite its tension-relieving properties (Zetin and Kramer)

  compulsive checking: light switches, gas taps, doors
  compulsive repeating: repeatedly touching an object, saying a prayer; entering a room a certain number of times to prevent harm befalling loved ones
  compulsive cleanliness: handwashing, frequent showers, repetitive cleaning of objects
  compulsive ordering of objects: eg. symmetry of bed linen

NB: after a long time, conscious resistance may wane if the subject yields to impulse

Related disorders

◆ Body dysmorphic disorder
◆ Trichotillomania
◆ Religious scrupulousness
◆ Urinary obsessions
◆ Compulsive facial picking

- Hoarding
- Hypochondriasis
- Paraphilias
- Anorexia nervosa (disputed)

Co-existing factors

- Major depression
- Simple or social phobia
- Separation anxiety
- Eating disorders
- Alcohol abuse / dependence
- Panic disorder
- Tourette's syndrome

Precipitation and presentation

- Behaviour is usually secretive and controlling
- Presentation usually occurs when
  - symptoms can no longer be hidden
  - frank depression supervenes
  - the family can no longer tolerate the behaviour
  - loss of friendships or job effectiveness
- Other precipitating factors
  - sexual and marital difficulties
  - pregnancy and delivery
  - illness or death of a near relative

Family history

- Family history of affective disorder (depression or anxiety disorder)
- Family history of substance abuse

Personal history

- Separation anxiety
- Mean age of onset around 22 years

Past medical history

- Affective disorder (depression or anxiety disorder)
- Substance abuse

Drug history

- Drugs used to treat OCD
  - clomipramine
  - selective serotonin reuptake inhibitors

Pre-morbid personality

- Personality traits
  - resistance to change or novelty
  - risk aversion
  - ambivalence
  - excessive devotion to work
  - magical thinking
  - hypermorality
  - perfectionism
- Personality disorder
  - avoidant
  - histrionic
  - dependent
  - mixed
- Substance misuse, including alcohol

Social circumstances

- Marriage

Psychosexual history

- Celibacy
- Marital problems
- Increased risk of separation or divorce (as in any psychiatric condition)

Mental state

- Evidence of compulsive behaviour (eg. raw hands from repeated washing)
- Affect
  - anxious

- Thoughts
  - guilt, helplessness, low self-esteem due to keeping the disease a secret
- Insight
  - present: the patient is very aware of the absurdity of the symptoms

Investigations

- Yale-Brown Obsessive-Compulsive checklist
- Blunted growth hormone response to IV clonidine
- Dexamethasone suppression test non-suppression
- Polysomnography
  - shortened REM latency, decreased total sleep time, decreased stage 4 sleep, decreased sleep efficiency, increased number of awakenings
- CT/MRI scans
  - orbital-frontal cortex, caudate and ventricular-brain ratio changes
- PET scan
  - increased activity bilaterally in the caudate nucleus and left orbital gyrus; increased frontal and cingulate abnormality
- Neuropsychology
  - spatial perceptual deficits similar to patients with frontal lobe lesions; age inappropriate synkinesias; abnormalities in fine motor co-ordination, involuntary and mirror movements

Management

- Biological
  - drugs acting on the serotonergic system
    clomipramine
    selective serotonin reuptake inhibitors
  - neurosurgery
    lesions in the cingulum and anterior capsule
- Psychological
  - education and support to the patient and the family
  - behavioural treatment
    exposure (systematic desensitisation)
    thought stopping
    homework assignments

✻   ✻   ✻   ✻   ✻

Just before you sat down to read this, did you shut the door? Perhaps someone is going to interrupt you. Wouldn't it be better just to check it really is closed, so they *really* know you don't want to be disturbed?

Have you just read the first paragraph again, after getting up to close the door? You did close it properly this time, didn't you? You're not sure. Well go and check it. I want your attention while you read this.

Good, you've finally closed that door. We can get on with it. What's that? You think that the door that you closed might have not quite caught the latch fully and may be coming open? OK. We don't want to be disturbed, so you better go and do it again. We could of course go on like for a long time. I am going to assume now that the door is at last closed — if you needed to shut it in the first place.

Checking is, in fact, a very sophisticated mental activity. Humans can detect that an error has occurred and put it right. We can even recall an act that we have done a few minutes ago, but may have done incorrectly. And we do not even need to think about it — suddenly, a thought pops into our mind, as though from nowhere. 'You did not lock the door properly'. We go back, find the door unlocked and lock it. We then get on with what we were doing when we were interrupted, secure in the knowledge that the door is locked. The matter is over and the error is corrected.

As with any mental mechanism, when it works correctly, it is very impressive. The trouble is that, as with anything else in the body, this is another of those systems that can go wrong. When it does, it is a peculiarly unpleasant sensation. The thought keeps coming into the person's mind that he or she has not done something properly. The person goes back and repeats the act. It is done, but a few seconds after leaving, the doubts come back. Of course, if this happens only two or three times — as it may well do to someone who is anxious or tired — and we can get on with the rest of the day, then that is irritating, but nothing more. If the doubt comes into the patient's head repeatedly and interrupts his or her ability to deal with other events for a matter of hours, then that is quite a different story. It can be recognised as a disorder.

It seems absurd to have such a symptom. Not only the observer, but the patient also is aware that the doubt is ludicrous. Despite this, he or she is powerless to resist the compulsion to check and check again that the eventuality has been dealt with, and if the doctor is unaware that this is the symptom of a psychiatric disorder, the patient can feel very stupid and embarrassed. It may be some time before the patient finds the stress of the repeated symptom greater than the fear of ridicule from the doctor.

A thought such as this, which comes spontaneously into the patient's mind and is recognised by the patient as being absurd, is called an **obsession** or an **obsessive thought**. It is a symptom found mainly in obsessive-compulsive disorder, although it can occur in depressive illness, or even in schizophrenia. There are various forms of obsessive symptom. It may be a thought, as mentioned above and may lead to constant doubt (**obsessive doubt**). It can be an obsessive idea, ie. an idea that is repeated again and again. It can be a constant anxiety about something terrible happening: the patient may be afraid being unable to prevent himself going to the kitchen, taking out a knife and harming himself or someone else. Such constant anxiety is referred to as an obsessive rumination. The result of such obsessions is that the patient takes a great deal of time to complete tasks or routines that others complete in minutes, for example, leaving the bedroom in the morning after making the bed - have the bed covers been aligned perfectly? This is referred to as **obsessive slowness**.

As with any other medical symptom, it is important to understand the definition. Many people use the term 'obsession' when they are describing somebody who is taking a great deal of interest in a pastime, ie. 'he is obsessed by football'. Psychiatrists do not have a monopoly over the use of language and they are not in a position to forbid colloquial usage. It is, therefore, important, when talking in a psychiatric context, to distinguish between the colloquial uses of the word 'obsession' and the technical use of the word as a psychiatric symptom.

The additional concern with respect to those who have these obsessional thoughts is that people act on them. Such an action is referred to as **compulsion**. There are many compulsive acts that people carry out in response to obsessive thoughts. They may feel a need to constantly check that light switches are switched off or doors are closed. They may feel particular anxiety about cleaning properly and respond by repeated handwashing until the hands are sore. An intense need for order and to repeatedly check the symmetry of the bed linen is a further symptom, or they may feel obliged to carry out an act that has some 'mystical' significance, such as touching the door on the way out to prevent a disaster occurring.

What help can be offered to such patients? Surprisingly, although there is a psychological explanation for these symptoms, considerable evidence exists to show that there is a biological basis to the disorder. In particular, dysfunction of the serotonergic systems in the brain has been found. Studies show that patients respond to the antidepressant clomipramine; this acts on the serotonergic system, but desipramine does not. Similarly, other drugs that enhance serotonergic transmission, SSRIs, seem to be of some benefit, and drug therapy is seen by many as the first choice treatment. Psychological therapies are usually directed at the symptoms rather than the underlying causes. Initially, making the diagnosis can help the patient to stop feeling quite so embarrassed about the symptoms. Secondly, the family can be advised and educated; this makes coping easier. Advising some patients to try 'thought stopping', in which they say 'stop' when the obsessive thought occurs, can help. If the symptom is part of an underlying disorder, such as depression, the obsessive-compulsive symptoms will ease as the underlying disorder improves.

Sources and further reading

Rapoport J (1989) *The Boy Who Couldn't Stop Washing: The experience and treatment of obsessive-compulsive disorder*. EP Dutton, New York

Tynes LL,White K,Steketee GS. (1990) Towards a new nosology of obsessive-compulsive disorder. *Comprehensive Psychiatry*, **31**(5):465-80 (September/October 1990)

Zetin M, Kramer MA (1992) Obsessive-compulsive disorder. *Hospital and Community Psychiatry*, **43**(7):689-699 (July 92)

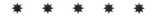

History of presenting complaint

The symptoms of obsessive-compulsive disorder are fairly constant, with factor analytic studies suggesting obsessions and checking; symmetry and ordering; cleanliness and washing; hoarding; thoughts of the past; and embarrassing behaviour often occurring together (Leckman *et al*, 1997, Khanna *et al*, 1990). Obsessional slowness seems to be secondary to recognised avoidance strategies or rituals (avoidance of disorder, lack of meticulousness, inexactness) (Ratnasuriya *et al*, 1991; Veale, 1993). For patients who reach secondary outpatient care, both behavioural and mental compulsions are often present (Foa *et al*, 1995).

It is important for the clinician to be clear about the definitions of the conditions, as there is a tendency for lay people to label anxieties and worries as obsessions, with a risk of over-diagnosis (Stein *et al*, 1997). Around 15% report life events (either desirable or undesirable) before the onset of the disorder; in men more than women, it is an undesirable life event (Lensi *et al*, 1996).

Family history

The incidence of OCD in first degree relatives of patients with OCD is around 10% compared with 2% in controls (Pauls *et al*, 1995). Patients often give a family history of psychiatric disorder, mainly depression: only in a small proportion (7.6%) is there a history of OCD in a first-degree relative (McKeon and Murray, 1987; Lensi *et al* 1996). There is, however, evidence of an increase in anxiety disorders in the first-degree relatives patients with OCD (Black *et al*, 1992).

Personal history

Males with OCD show a higher incidence of perinatal trauma (Lensi *et al*, 1996). With peak onset in the early 30s, many men work prior to onset of the disorder; many women are housewives or unemployed (Lensi *et al*, 1996).

Past medical history

There may be an association with head injury (Drummond and Gravestock, 1988).

Past psychiatric history

There is a relationship with Gilles de la Tourette syndrome. In one study, subjects with comorbid Tourette's syndrome had significantly more violent, sexual and symmetrical obsessions, and more touching, blinking, counting, and self-damaging compulsions, compared with a group with obsessive-compulsive disorder alone, who had more obsessions connected with dirt or germs and more cleaning compulsions (George *et al*, 1993). There is co-morbidity in 50% of patients with generalised anxiety disorder, panic disorder and depressive illness, but not bipolar affective disorder (Lensi *et al*, 1996; Nelson and Rice, 1997) and substance misuse (Nelson and Rice, 1997). There is also a comorbidity of around 7.5% with schizophrenia (Eisen *et al*, 1997) and a comorbidity of 12% with body dysmorphic disorder (Simeon *et al*, 1995). A comorbidity of 37% with eating disorders exists (Thiel *et al*, 1995).

Drug history

Evidence suggests that symptoms of OCD are induced or exacerbated by clozapine (Eales and Layeni, 1994) and nefazodone (Sofuoglu and Debattista, 1996).

Pre-morbid personality

There does not seem to be a relationship between obsessive personality and obsessive-compulsive disorder (Baer *et al*, 1990; Black *et al*, 1993). Neither has a specific personality trait been observed, although a mixed personality disorder with avoidant, dependent, histrionic and passive-aggressive features was most commonly observed in the obsessive-compulsive group (Joffe *et al*, 1988; Baer *et al*, 1990).

The presence of traits of personality disorder should be sought as there is evidence that patients with of schizotypal, borderline and avoidant personality disorders, or traits of more than one additional personality disorder, have a poorer treatment outcome in treatment with clomipramine (Baer *et al*, 1992). Patients with OCD exhibit low levels of alcohol and benzodiazepine abuse (Lensi *et al*, 1996), but abuse of cocaine may induce obsessive symptoms (Satel and McDougle, 1991).

Social circumstances

Fifty percent of women and 25% of men get married (Lensi *et al*, 1996). Rather than being rejected, many patients remain with their parents or spouse, who accommodate the patient's symptoms by modifying personal and family routines. However, attitudes of relatives may show a rejecting attitude towards the patient (Calvocoressi *et al*, 1995). In many marriages, there is evidence of distress in the spouses, which is not alleviated when OCD symptoms improve in response to treatment (Emmelkamp *et al*, 1990).

Mental state examination

Insight is generally regarded as necessary to the diagnosis, but field trials suggest that this is not always fully intact, in that patients do not always regard their symptoms as unreasonable or excessive (Foa *et al*, 1995). There was no resistance to compulsive behaviour in 12% of one group of patients, and more bizarre beliefs were less likely to be considered irrational: neither of these features reduced the likelihood of response to treatment (Lelliott *et al*, 1988).

A number of neurological soft signs have been observed in OCD, such as signs of central nervous system dysfunction in obsessive-compulsive disorder. Hollander *et al* (1990) describe abnormalities in fine motor coordination, involuntary and mirror movements and visuospatial function, correlating with the severity of obsessions.

Management

Drug treatment

There is evidence that drugs acting on the serotonergic system (selective serotonin re-uptake inhibitors, clomipramine) are effective in easing the symptoms of patients with OCD (The Clomipramine Collaborative Study Group, 1991; Zohar *et al*, 1996). In contrast, tricyclic antidepressants that are more active on noradrenergic pathways, such as desipramine (Barr *et al*, 1997) and monoamine oxidase inhibitors (Jenike *et al*, 1997) do not. Changes in the function of the caudate can be shown in association with successful response to clomipramine (Benkelfat *et al*, 1990) and fluoxetine (Baxter *et al*, 1992).

In a study looking at the possibility of a dose-response to sertraline, the evidence was unclear. Doses of 50mg/day, 100mg/day and 200mg/day were more effective than placebo, but 50mg and 200mg showed better response than 100mg/day (Griest *et al*, 1995). After successful treatment, there may be a need for maintenance treatment, as there is some evidence that patients, treated successfully with clomipramine, relapse after drug discontinuation (Pato *et al*, 1988). Addition of lithium and l-tryptophan to clomipramine has been tried in refractory patients (Rasmussen, 1984).

Neuroleptics do not seem to be of benefit in obsessive-compulsive disorder, either on their own or as an adjunct to pharmacological agents acting on the serotonergic system. They are only found to be of benefit when there is a symptom of a related disorder, such as the presence of a tic (McDougle *et al*, 1994). A review of drug treatment can be found in Piccinelli *et al* (1995).

Maintenance ECT has been tried in refractory patients (Husain *et al*, 1993) and there is evidence that ventromedial frontal leucotomy (Irle *et al*, 1998) or cingulotomy (Baer *et al*, 1995) can be helpful as a treatment of last resort in highly refractory patients.

Psychological treatments

Exposure and ritual prevention have been shown to be effective treatments, particularly in those who are most compliant in the first week of treatment (De Araujo *et al*, 1996). Evidence suggests that it is these treatments and not non-specific aspects of the therapy process, such as general anxiety management techniques (eg. relaxation) that lead to the improvements (Marks, 1981; Lindsay *et al*, 1997). However, there is evidence that greater initial severity of complaints and co-existent depression separately predict poor outcome of treatment of compulsive behaviour with *in vivo* exposure and response prevention. In addition to these factors, poorer motivation and dissatisfaction with the therapeutic relationship predict poorer outcome of treatment of obsessive fear (Keijsers *et al*, 1994). Successful response to exposure and response prevention is associated with changes demonstrable by PET in the caudate nucleus (Baxter *et al*, 1992; Schwartz *et al*, 1996).

Cognitive therapy has been tried as a treatment for OCD, but a recent review (James and Blackburn, 1995) concluded that there are very few studies, with little evidence of improvement when cognitive therapy is added to existing techniques.

The majority of patients (87% in one study, Orloff *et al* 1994) will have responded to treatment within one year. For some, response is maintained or even increased over one to three years, although no predictors of clinical features or treatment package could be determined.

References

Baer L, Jenike MA, Ricciardi JN 2nd *et al* (1990 Standardized assessment of personality disorders in obsessive-compulsive disorder. *Arch Gen Psychiatry* 47: 826–30

Baer L, Jenike MA, Black DW *et al* (1992) Effect of axis II diagnoses on treatment outcome with clomipramine in 55 patients with obsessive-compulsive disorder. *Arch Gen Psychiatry* **49**: 862–6

Baer L, Rauch SL, Ballantine HT Jr *et al* (1995) Cingulotomy for intractable obsessive-compulsive disorder. Prospective long-term follow-up of 18 patients. *Arch Gen Psychiatry* **52**: 384–92

Barr LC, Goodman WK, Anand A, McDougle CJ, Price LH (1997) Addition of desipramine to serotonin reuptake inhibitors in treatment-resistant obsessive-compulsive disorder. *Am J Psychiatry* **154**: 1293–5

Baxter LR Jr, Schwartz JM, Bergman KS *et al* (1992) Caudate glucose metabolic rate changes with both drug and behavior therapy for obsessive-compulsive disorder. *Arch Gen Psychiatry* **49**: 681–9

Benkelfat C, Nordahl TE, Semple WE, King AC, Murphy DL, Cohen RM (1990) Local cerebral glucose metabolic rates in obsessive-compulsive disorder. Patients treated with clomipramine. *Arch Gen Psychiatry* **47**: 840–8

Black DW, Noyes R Jr, Goldstein RB, Blum N (1992) A family study of obsessive-compulsive disorder. *Arch Gen Psychiatry* **49**: 362–8

Black DW, Noyes R Jr, Pfohl B, Goldstein RB, Blum N (1993) Personality disorder in obsessive-compulsive volunteers, well comparison subjects, and their first-degree relatives. *Am J Psychiatry* **150**: 1226–32

Calvocoressi L, Lewis B, Harris M *et al* (1995) Family accommodation in obsessive-compulsive disorder. *Am J Psychiatry* **152**: 441–3

The Clomipramine Collaborative Study Group (1991) Clomipramine in the treatment of patients with obsessive-compulsive disorder. *Arch Gen Psychiatry* **48**: 730–8

De Araujo LA, Ito LM, Marks IM (1996) Early compliance and other factors predicting outcome of exposure for obsessive-compulsive disorder. *Br J Psychiatry* **169**: 747–52

Drummond LM, Gravestock S (1988) Delayed emergence of obsessive-compulsive neurosis following head injury: case report and review of its theoretical implications. *Br J Psychiatry* **153**: 839–42

Eales MJ, Layeni AO (1994) Exacerbation of obsessive-compulsive symptoms associated with clozapine. *Br J Psychiatry* **164**: 687–8

Eisen JL, Beer DA, Pato MT, Venditto TA, Rasmussen SA (1997) Obsessive-compulsive disorder in patients with schizophrenia or schizoaffective disorder. *Am J Psychiatry* **154**: 271–3

Emmelkamp PMG, de Haan E, Hoogduin CAL (1990) Marital adjustment and obsessive-compulsive disorder. *Br J Psychiatry* **156**: 55–60

Foa EB, Kozak MJ, Goodman WK, Hollander E, Jenike MA, Rasmussen SA (1995) DSM-IV field trial: obsessive-compulsive disorder. *Am J Psychiatry* **152**: 90–6

George MS, Trimble MR, Ring HA, Sallee FR, Robertson MM (1993) Obsessions in obsessive-compulsive disorder with and without Gilles de la Tourette's syndrome. *Am J Psychiatry* **150**: 93–7

Greist J, Chouinard G, DuBoff E *et al* (1995) Double-blind parallel comparison of three dosages of sertraline and placebo in outpatients with obsessive-compulsive disorder. *Arch Gen Psychiatry* **52**: 289–95

Hollander E, Schiffman E, Cohen B *et al* (1990) Signs of central nervous system dysfunction in obsessive-compulsive disorder. *Arch Gen Psychiatry* **47**: 27–32

Husain MM, Lewis SF, Thornton WL (1993) Maintenance ECT for refractory obsessive-compulsive disorder. *Am J Psychiatry* **150**: 1899–900

Irle E, Exner C, Thielen K, Weniger G, Ruther E (1998) Obsessive-compulsive disorder and ventromedial frontal lesions: clinical and neuropsychological findings. *Am J Psychiatry* **155**: 255–63

James IA, Blackburn I-M (1995) Cognitive therapy with obsessive-compulsive disorder. *Br J Psychiatry* **166**: 444–50

Jenike MA, Baer L, Minichiello WE, Rauch SL, Buttolph ML (1997) Placebo-controlled trial of fluoxetine and phenelzine for obsessive-compulsive disorder. *Am J Psychiatry* **154**: 1261–4

Joffe RT, Swinson RP, Regan JJ (1988) Personality features of obsessive-compulsive disorder. *Am J Psychiatry* **145**: 1127–9

Keijsers GPJ, Hoogduin CAL, Schaap CPDR (1994) Predictors of treatment outcome in the behavioural treatment of obsessive-compulsive disorder. *Br J Psychiatry* **165**: 781–6

Khanna S, Kaliaperumal VG, Channabasavanna SM (1990) Clusters of obsessive-compulsive phenomena in obsessive-compulsive disorder. *Br J Psychiatry* **156**: 51–4

Leckman JF, Grice DE, Boardman J *et al* (1997) Symptoms of obsessive-compulsive disorder. *Am J Psychiatry* **154**: 911–7

Lelliott PT, Noshirvani HF, Basoglu M, Marks IM, Monteiro WO (1988) Obsessive-compulsive beliefs and treatment outcome. *Psychol Med* **18**: 697–702

Lensi P, Cassano PB, Correddu G, Ravagli S, Kunovac JL, Akiskal HS (1996) Obsessive-compulsive disorder. Familial-developmental history, symptomatology, co-morbidity and course with special reference to gender-related differences. *Br J Psychiatry* **169**: 101–7

Lindsay M, Crino R, Andrews G (1997) Controlled trial of exposure and response prevention in obsessive-compulsive disorder. *Br J Psychiatry* **171**: 135–9

Marks IM (1981) Review of behavioral psychotherapy, I: Obsessive-compulsive disorders. *Am J Psychiatry* **138**: 584–92

McDougle CJ, Goodman WK, Leckman JF, Lee NC, Heninger GR, Price LH (1994) Haloperidol addition in fluvoxamine-refractory obsessive-compulsive disorder. A double-blind, placebo-controlled study in patients with and without tics. *Arch Gen Psychiatry* **51**: 302–8

McKeon P, Murray R (1987) Familial aspects of obsessive-compulsive neurosis. *Br J Psychiatry* **151**: 528–34

Nelson E, Rice J (1997) Stability of diagnosis of obsessive-compulsive disorder in the Epidemiologic Catchment Area study. *Am J Psychiatry* **154**: 826–31

Orloff LM, Battle MA *et al* (1994) Long-term follow-up of 85 patients with obsessive-compulsive disorder. *Am J Psychiatry* **151**: 441–2

Pato MT, Zohar-Kadouch R, Zohar J, Murphy DL (1988) Return of symptoms after discontinuation of clomipramine in patients with obsessive-compulsive disorder. *Am J Psychiatry* **145**: 1521–5

Pauls DL, Alsobrook JP 2nd, Goodman W, Rasmussen S, Leckman JF (1995) A family study of obsessive-compulsive disorder. *Am J Psychiatry* **152**: 76–84

Piccinelli M, Pini S, Bellantuono C, Wilkinson G (1995) Efficacy of drug treatment in obsessive-compulsive disorder. A meta-analytic review. *Br J Psychiatry* **166**: 424–43

Rasmussen SA (1984) Lithium and tryptophan augmentation in clomipramine-resistant obsessive-compulsive disorder. *Am J Psychiatry* **141**: 1283–5

Ratnasuriya RH, Marks IM, Forshaw DM, Hymas NFS (1991) Obsessive slowness revisited. *Br J Psychiatry* **159**: 273–4

Satel SL, McDougle CJ (1991) Obsessions and compulsions associated with cocaine abuse. *Am J Psychiatry* **148**: 947

Schwartz JM, Stoessel PW, Baxter LR Jr, Martin KM, Phelps ME (1996) Systematic changes in cerebral glucose metabolic rate after successful behavior modification treatment of obsessive-compulsive disorder. *Arch Gen Psychiatry* **53**: 109–13

Simeon D, Hollander E, Stein DJ, Cohen L, Aronowitz B (1995) Body dysmorphic disorder in the DSM-IV field trial for obsessive-compulsive disorder. *Am J Psychiatry* **152**: 1207–9

Sofuoglu M, Debattista C (1996) Development of obsessive symptoms during nefazodone treatment. *Am J Psychiatry* **153**: 577–8

Stein MB, Forde DR, Anderson G, Walker JR (1997) Obsessive-compulsive disorder in the community: an epidemiologic survey with clinical reappraisal. *Am J Psychiatry* **154**: 1120–6

Thiel A, Broocks A, Ohlmeier M, Jacoby GE, Schussler G (1995) Obsessive-compulsive disorder among patients with anorexia nervosa and bulimia nervosa. *Am J Psychiatry* **152**: 72–5

Veale D (1993) Classification and treatment of obsessional slowness. *Br J Psychiatry* **162**: 198–203

Zohar J, Judge R, and the OCD Paroxetine Study Investigators (1996) Paroxetine versus clomipramine in the treatment of obsessive-compulsive disorder. *Br J Psychiatry* **169**: 468–74

9

Personality disorder (Antisocial)

History

1. Symptoms

- Failure to make loving relationships
- Impulsive actions
- Lack of guilt / remorse
- Failure to learn from adverse experiences
- Manipulative behaviour
- Difficulties present since adolescence

2. Associated features

- Depression
- Anxiety
- Deliberate self harm
- Family history
- Aggressive behaviour of father/parent
- Marital disharmony
- Lack of adequate parenting
- Other members of the family abuse alcohol or have received psychiatric treatment for depression

Personal history

- Separation from mother
- Truanting from school
- Aggressive behaviour towards other children
- Fire-raising, torture of animals, enuresis (Hellman's triad)
- Mixing with delinquents
- Abuse of substances
- Unstable work record, marked by frequent dismissals

Past medical history

- Alcohol-related problems

Past psychiatric history

- Conduct disorder
- Many brief psychiatric admissions, often with the patient discharging himself after 1-2 days
- Parasuicide
- Deliberate self-harm, especially with razor blades (releases tension)
- Depressive episodes
  - often a clearl response to a particular adverse circumstance
- Anxiety disorder
- Substance abuse
  - alcohol, heroin, methadone, cocaine etc, polydrug abuse
- Previous episode of head injury
- May have consulted many therapists, for brief periods of time, and found none helpful

Drug history

- Anxiolytics, especially in high doses
- Antidepressants

Pre-morbid personality

- Cold
- Callous
- No friends
- Detached
- Humourless
- Failing to accept authority

Forensic history

- Includes convictions for Grievous Bodily Harm
- Prison sentences
- Juvenile convictions
- Smokes cigarettes and may abuse drugs

Social circumstances

◆ Frequent changes of accommodation

Psychosexual history

◆ No partners
◆ Many partners, brief relationships, often violent and ended by violence

Mental state examination

Appearance and behaviour

◆ Very demanding patient
◆ May be very threatening to the interviewer
◆ May appear very anxious or tense
◆ Linear scars on forearms (or other parts of body), usually self-inflicted, often by razor blades
◆ Unkempt
◆ Untidy
◆ Tattoo marks

Mood

◆ Depressed
◆ Anxious

Affect

◆ Depressed
◆ Anxious
◆ Tense

Speech

◆ Threatening content
◆ Manipulative content
◆ Often tries the technique of splitting (will report to one person the alleged comments of another)
◆ A tendency to blame others, even when it is more likely to be his/her own fault
◆ Lack of empathy (expects others to see his point of view, but will not acknowledge the other person's point of view)
◆ Tells falsehoods or lies

Thoughts

- Often are of suicidal intent that may be very strong; usually because angry with the world
- No clear paranoid ideas
- No low self-esteem
- No guilt: tendency to be angry with others and to see self as an innocent victim
- Pessimism about the future

Experiences

- No hallucinations or first rank symptoms

Cognition

- Intact

Insight

- Externalization of locus of control, so that does not believe that is responsible for own misfortunes; often very aware of neurotic complaints and insistent about them.

Management

It is important to try to avoid a judgmental attitude. This is particularly difficult when the patient is making you feel uncomfortable. The distress that the patient presents at times of crisis is genuine, even if the cause of the crisis and the patient's inappropriate responses seem ridiculous.

- Assessment of the problem
  - ❑ informant history

    parent
    spouse or partner
    probation officer, including criminal record
    medical notes
    solicitor or barrister
    legal depositions in court cases
    persuading the patient to write his/her life history
    factors that provoke aggressiveness
- Exclude organic cause
  - ❑ focal or diffuse brain disorder
  - ❑ toxic or metabolic
  - ❑ ictal disorder
  - ❑ EEG
- Assess co-existent psychiatric disorder

- Avoid benzodiazepines (risk of dependence; risk of disinhibiting effect releasing aggressive behaviour)
- Set limits
  - when talking to the patient about something distressing, gently hand the responsibility for his actions back to him, while offering to support him if he makes a prudent choice
  - aim for consistency between professionals: good communication is crucial

    never blame another professional simply on the basis of an uncorroborated complaint by the patient

    never accept an alleged comment that the patient is attributing to another professional without checking it: if you cannot, simply say that you can neither accept nor reject that this is what the other person said, and do not act on such an alleged comment.
- Individual psychotherapy
  - aim is usually supportive rather than dynamic
  - psychiatrist; CPN; social worker; probation officer
  - counselling
  - practical help, ie. learn to recognise precipitants of aggressive behaviour and their modification
  - social skills training
  - avoid dependence on the therapist
  - recognise when support is not providing any benefit and terminate the sessions
- Small group psychotherapy
  - with other patients with the same diagnosis; not patients with other diagnoses
- therapeutic community; milieu therapy
- Grendon prison
- Court reports are often requested
  - assess what is likely to have happened in the alleged incident
  - look for any genuine psychiatric reason that the court might take into consideration
  - do not be swayed in favour of, or against the patient because of his own overt manipulation. The psychiatrist is not there to try and find an excuse for a person, who knew what he/she were doing, to avoid prison or other consequences of his/her actions. However, you can make statements that might be helpful to the patient, if they are medically valid
  - if you feel that there is nothing that you can offer that would help the patient cope better in future, and if you feel that there is no psychiatric treatment at your disposal that would help the patient, it is your duty to say so
  - **never** let a solicitor dictate to you what he wants you to say. Draw your own medical conclusions, and then ask the solicitor if your opinion will help his client. If not, do not let him change your views

❑ your job as an expert witness is always to assist the court, by giving a valid psychiatric assessment, whoever asks you to prepare the report, and irrespective of which side is paying you. In contrast, it is the duty of the solicitor or barrister to do everything he can to present his client's case in the best possible light.

✳   ✳   ✳   ✳   ✳

Perhaps the most contentious diagnosis in psychiatry is that of personality disorder. In disorders, such as schizophrenia, where patients have grossly abnormal mental experiences, ie. hearing the voices of people who are not there, few would say that there is not something seriously wrong with their mental function. In personality disorder, features do not always seem to be abnormal. For example, anger is a normal, psychological function, so if a person is angry and does not control it, why should he/she not be held responsible for his/her subsequent actions? Society recognises that some of these people are different and may need psychiatric help. Is this a medical condition? There is no definitive answer and this causes continuing confusion. Society expects a definite answer and is unwilling to accept the professional's failure to provide one.

Let us attempt to clarify the situation. It appears there is a group of people who have problems that can, in effect, be attributed to their personality. Personality is a psychological attribute and as such is of legitimate concern to the psychiatrist when it seems to malfunction. However, an understanding of a psychological attribute does not mean it is necessarily a justification for removing a person's responsibility for his actions. Hence the arguments with moral philosophers, lawyers, criminologists, etc. To illustrate, without suggesting that a diagnosis of personality disorder should be made, consider the behaviour of Eric Cantona, the footballer who played for Manchester United. Although a gifted player, he had on several occasions hit other players in the course of the game and been sent off the field of play. On 25 January 1995, he was sent off while playing at Crystal Palace in London. As he walked from the field, Crystal Palace fans were abusing him. At one point he responded to the abuse by assaulting one of the fans. We can understand the provocation, and Eric Cantona's anger, but that does not absolve him of responsibility for his assault, and he later received a conviction in the English courts for this offence. (He was also banned from playing by the English Football Association. Following this, his behaviour on the field was greatly improved)

Given the complexity of the term, what is meant by **personality** and what is meant by the term **personality disorder?** Experts are unable to agree a definition of personality, but it is generally acceptable to consider personality to be a set of behaviours that a person habitually uses in response to recurring situations. For example, should a cup be accidentally dropped and broken, one person might swear angrily, another may shrug it off and a third will laugh. Although responses vary on different occasions, it would not be surprising to find that the three people responded in the same way in other frustrating, accidental situations. It is not invariable, but individuals do seem to have a preferred response for dealing with repeated situations.

If personality represents habitual actions, then a disorder of personality must indicate when those habitual actions are unhelpful to the person and cause problems. If a person responds to provocation by swearing, there may be no consequences. If a person responds to the same provocation by committing an assault, he may end up in prison. The situation is the same, but the response is different.

Not all responses are violent and there are various types of personality problems that may lead to the involvement of a doctor. A patient may be very rigid in his lifestyle, ie. very strict in his routine and resistant to changes. Such a person would be described as having an **obsessional** or **anankastic** personality. He might be particularly sensitive to the comments and criticisms of others, and be referred to as having a **paranoid** personality. Contact with others may be limited and he may appear aloof, living in a solitary world, but without reaching the criteria for a diagnosis of schizophrenia. Such a person could be described as having a **schizoid** personality. There may be a tendency to dramatise relatively trivial situations and constantly seek the appreciation of others. This could be described as having a **histrionic** personality.

A person who feels a need to be dependent on others and who expects others to be responsible for his/her actions could be described as having a **dependent** personality. An individual who is very anxious about being with other people, especially if there is a risk of criticism, is defined as having an **anxious** or **avoidant** personality.

The list does not cover the whole personality structure; only those that are regularly brought to the attention of psychiatrists and other doctors. It has been formally described in the World Health Organisation's International Classification of Diseases, 10th Edition (ICD-10). It should be noted that these are structures of personality. The person is regarded as having a **disorder** of personality when the personality traits lead the person, or people associated with him/her, to suffer repeated physical, psychological or social harm.

The list would be incomplete if we fail to mention **the emotionally unstable** personality disorder. Symptoms include: a failure to plan ahead; responding to the environment with impulsive outbursts that show no regard for the consequences. And the **dissocial** or **antisocial** personality disorder, in which the person has a callous disregard for the feelings of others, disregards social obligations and rules, has a low frustration tolerance accompanied by aggressive outbursts. This followed by a complete lack of remorse and a disposition to blame others. These latter two types are the most unpleasant to deal with, and when a patient is described as having a personality disorder without further clarification of the type of personality disorder, it is usually taken to mean one of these two.

One aspect of the label, **personality disorder**, is the expectation that it will be resistant to change. In psychiatry this is important, as we try to distinguish repeated behaviours that have continued since adolescence — when the personality is thought to become fixed — from repeated behaviours that are of recent origin, and suggestive of a disease process or illness. Thus, many people will observe, in their relatives, a personality change in the early stages of depressive, hypomanic or schizophrenic illness, dementia, or after a serious head injury — suggesting a greater degree of brain damage than originally diagnosed.

In patients with personality disorder, the signs may have been there for some time. For example, if a patient has the dissocial personality, antisocial behaviour may have occurred at school and at work (if the person stayed in a job for any length of time). It may have led to the break-up of relationships and to convictions for violent crime and periods of time in prison. The constant level of tension may have been self-medicated with alcohol or other drugs, especially benzodiazepines, although both of these can have a disinhibiting effect and lead the person into more trouble from further aggressive outbursts. The patient is, perhaps surprisingly, rarely unwilling to give all this information to a doctor.

The management of personality disorder involves recognition not only of the condition and an understanding of its psychology, but also a recognition by the therapist that the patient (and those around him) are suffering much more than the doctor trying to manage it. With an understanding of the condition, the doctor should approach the situation in as sympathetic a manner as possible.

This is not to deny the doctor's right to protect himself or herself from a potentially violent patient, or to disarm manipulations by a manipulative patient. No doctor should collude with the patient by using the presence of a personality disorder as a false justification for excusing a criminal act, for example, by writing a biased court report on behalf of the patient. Neither should the doctor submit to other questionable demands from the patient arising out of the personality disorder. The doctor will need to set limits to the behaviours that can be tolerated and to compliance of requests from the patient. This will provide a structure that prevents the doctor from having to reject the patient in most circumstances. With such clearly defined limits set, and accepted by the patient (in practice, if not in word), it may be possible for the doctor to help the patient look at his or her unhelpful behaviours and, perhaps very slowly, make changes.

Personality disorder is a diagnosis that is distinct from almost all other diagnoses in medicine in that it frequently evokes emotional rather than scientific discussions. Perhaps the wisest initial approach by the clinician is to recognise that there will be frequent presentations by people who show a number of behaviours that have been defined in the major diagnostic classifications (ICD-10 and DSM-IV) as **personality disorders**. The role of the clinician is to:

- diagnose the presence of the condition, as defined in the major psychiatric classificatory systems
- use the knowledge of the condition to make some sense of why the patient is presenting with a problem at the current time (assuming that the presenting problem is related to personality)
- provide some suggestions that may alleviate the immediate circumstance or problem
- assist the patient to make longer-term changes, either in strategies used or (if possible) in cognitive set, that will reduce the frequency of crises arising and relieve the intensity of distress being experienced.

This group of patients do not respond easily to therapeutic interventions, and their behaviour is often demanding, hostile and, at times, physically threatening. There is a strong temptation to reject such patients with therapeutic nihilism, such as 'it is all their own fault'; 'I will not treat a violent patient', or 'they do not have a (real) mental illness'. It may be suggested that such an attitude is unnecessarily negative. The solution for the clinician is to recognise the problem, ensure his or her own safety and be aware of what help can be offered, or, conversely, whether it has passed beyond clinical relevance. The clinician should not only be sympathetic to the plight and the distress of the patient, but also be clear about the difference between sympathetically understanding the condition and making excuses for a patient's antisocial behaviour. The clinician should avoid any tendency to do this.

It is the opinion of a body of clinicians (including the author) that antisocial personality disorder is a chronic, psychological condition, amenable to various forms of psychological intervention, in which changes for the better can, in a number of cases, occur slowly over time. However, many other clinicians do not hold this view.

History of presenting complaint

The features of antisocial personality disorder (psychopathic personality disorder) have been disputed. Attempts have been made to categorise the various features into discrete pathological clusters (Gunn and Robertson, 1976; Reich and Thompson, 1987; Hume, 1990), but current classification is essentially operational.

Presentation will often be precipitated by a crisis, such as a fight, involvement with the police, or parasuicidal intention or behaviour, or with a complaint of unrelieved distress ('resistant depression').

Family history

People who show antisocial behaviour often come from families in which there is assaultive behaviour (Pfeffer *et al*, 1983). The genetic contribution is uncertain. A recent twin study concluded that symptoms of antisocial behaviour in children could be accounted for entirely by shared environment (Thapar and McGuffin, 1996). However, a recent adoption study has shown that a biologic background of antisocial personality disorder made an independent contribution to increased adolescent aggressiveness, conduct disorder and adult antisocial behaviours, in addition to an effect of adverse adoptive home environment (Cadoret *et al*, 1995).

It would appear that the children of alcoholics have higher lifetime rates of antisocial symptoms (Mathew *et al*, 1993), although it appears that it is not the parental alcoholism, but a history of physical abuse that is connected with antisocial symptoms in the child (Pollock *et al*, 1990).

There is also evidence that harsh, aggressive, explosive and inconsistent parenting contributes to adolescent antisocial behaviour. Siblings who do not receive such treatment from the parent appear not to show such antisocial behaviour (Reiss *et al*, 1995).

Personal history

Evidence from earlier studies suggests that antisocial behaviour in adulthood is almost always preceded by antisocial behaviour in childhood. However, most antisocial children do not become antisocial adults. Adult antisocial behaviour is better predicted by childhood behaviour than by family background, social class of rearing or current social class (Robins, 1978). There is longitudinal evidence that children who were under-controlled — this includes children who are impulsive, restless and distractible — at age three years, were more likely to meet criteria for antisocial personality disorder, attempt suicide and (if boys) have alcohol-related problems than comparison subjects (Caspi *et al*, 1996). There is some evidence that many patients who develop personality disorder in adolescence have slightly higher likelihood of a history of behavioural difficulties, such as conduct disorder in childhood (Bernstein *et al*, 1996). Adolescents with a diagnosis of conduct disorder and substance abuse go on to develop a diagnosis of antisocial personality disorder in a majority of cases (Myers *et al*, 1998; Eppright *et al*, 1993).

Hellman's triad of enuresis, firesetting and cruelty to animals (Hellman and Blackman, 1966) and hyperactivity are risk factors for the development of antisocial personality disorder and drug abuse (Mannuzza *et al*, 1998). It has also been suggested that childhood abuse or victimisation increases the likelihood of a diagnosis of antisocial personality disorder (Luntz and Widom, 1994).

Past medical history

There may be marked personality change following a serious head injury, which should be sought as a differential diagnosis. There is a strong association between antisocial personality disorder and substance use. Among intravenous drug users, antisocial personality disorder has been suggested as a major risk factor for contracting HIV (Brooner *et al*, 1993).

Past psychiatric history

The patient with a personality disorder often seems tense, anxious and distressed. Although such patients can develop psychotic illness, presentations to services frequently arise as a result of maladaptive attempts to cope with distress, such as parasuicide, other self-harm, such as self-wounding or self cutting (Tantam and Whittaker, 1992), or substance abuse. Other reasons include presentation with a resistant mood disorder, such as anxiety or depression.

Drug history

Many patients with antisocial personality disorder persuade their doctors to prescribe CNS depressant drugs, such as benzodiazepines in high doses (eg. 100mg daily) or methadone (if opiate-dependent) to alleviate feelings of tension.

Pre-morbid personality

Many patients have co-morbid substance use of opiates and/or stimulants. In many cases, there is evidence that antisocial personality traits precede drug-taking (Rounsaville *et al*, 1991; Brooner *et al*, 1997).

Social circumstances

A significant proportion of patients with antisocial personality disorder are involved in partner violence (Danielson *et al*, 1998) and the presence of antisocial personality disorder is a risk factor among women for committing homicide (Eronen, 1995).

A number of people with antisocial personality disorder are homeless. There is evidence that the number of antisocial symptoms among the homeless correlates with the number of conduct disorder symptoms and that the symptoms of antisocial disorder precede homelessness, suggesting that antisocial personality disorder may play a part in the aetiology of homelessness. This is not true of the reverse, ie. homelessness does not seem to cause antisocial behaviour (North *et al*, 1993).

Mental state examination

There is evidence that an ability to form a therapeutic alliance with the therapist is a good prognostic factor in patients with antisocial personality disorder (Gerstley *et al*, 1989).

Management

Data are lacking in this area, but there is some evidence that improvement in the core symptoms of personality disorder can be effected by a period of admission to a therapeutic community (Dolan *et al*, 1997). Care should be taken in the selection of patients to maximise efficacy (Norton and Hinshelwood, 1996).

In less intensive settings, where additional symptoms of borderline personality disorder are present, there may be some benefit from brief adaptive psychotherapy or short-term dynamic therapy (Winston *et al*, 1994) or supportive psychotherapy (Holmes, 1995). Attempts have been made to use medication to attenuate feelings of aggression in patients with antisocial personality disorder, such as fluoxetine (Coccaro and Kavoussi, 1997), lithium or carbamazepine (Greenberg, 1986). Treatments that may have some efficacy in reducing deliberate self-harm include: problem-solving therapy, provision of an emergency contact card, depot flupenthixol and dialectical behaviour therapy (Hawton *et al*, 1998).

References

Bernstein DP, Cohen P, Skodol A, Bezirganian S, Brook JS (1996) Childhood antecedents of adolescent personality disorders. *Am J Psychiatry* 153: 907–13

Brooner RK, Greenfield L, Schmidt CW, Bigelow GE (1993) Antisocial personality disorder and HIV infection among intravenous drug abusers. *Am J Psychiatry* **150**: 53–8

RK, King VL, Kidorf M, Schmidt CW Jr, Bigelow GE (1997) Psychiatric and substance use comorbidity among treatment-seeking opioid abusers. *Arch Gen Psychiatry* **54**: 71–80

Cadoret RJ, Yates WR, Troughton E, Woodworth G, Stewart MA (1995) Genetic-environmental interaction in the genesis of aggressivity and conduct disorders. *Arch Gen Psychiatry* **52**: 916–24

Caspi A, Moffitt TE, Newman DL, Silva PA (1996) Behavioral observations at age 3 years predict adult psychiatric disorders. Longitudinal evidence from a birth cohort. *Arch Gen Psychiatry* **53**: 1033–9

Coccaro EF, Kavoussi RJ (1997) Fluoxetine and impulsive aggressive behavior in personality-disordered subjects. *Arch Gen Psychiatry* **54**: 1081–8

Danielson KK, Moffitt TE, Caspi A, Silva PA (1998) Comorbidity between abuse of an adult and DSM-III-R mental disorders: evidence from an epidemiological study. *Am J Psychiatry* **155**: 131–3

Dolan B, Warren F, Norton K (1997) Change in borderline symptoms one year after therapeutic community treatment for severe personality disorder. *Br J Psychiatry* **171**: 274–9

Eppright TD, Kashani JH, Robison BD, Reid JC (1993) Comorbidity of conduct disorder and personality disorders in an incarcerated juvenile population. *Am J Psychiatry* **150**: 1233–6

Eronen M (1995) Mental disorders and homicidal behavior in female subjects. *Am J Psychiatry* **152**: 1216–8

Gerstley L, McLellan AT, Alterman AI, Woody GE, Luborsky L, Prout M (1989) Ability to form an alliance with the therapist: a possible marker of prognosis for patients with antisocial personality disorder. *Am J Psychiatry* **146**: 508–12

Greenberg WM (1986) Sedative or antimanic effects of carbamazepine and treatment of behavioral dyscontrol. *Am J Psychiatry* **143**: 1486–7

Gunn J, Robertson G (1976) Psychopathic personality: a conceptual problem. *Psychol Med* **6**: 631–4

Hawton K, Arensman E, Townsend E *et al* (1998) Deliberate self-harm: systematic review of efficacy of psychosocial and pharmacological treatments in preventing repetition. *Br Med J* **317**: 441–7

Hellman DS, Blackman N (1966) Enuresis, firesetting and cruelty to animals: a triad predictive of adult crime. *Am J Psychiatry* **122**: 1431–5

Holmes J (1995) Supportive psychotherapy. The search for positive meanings. *Br J Psychiatry* **167**: 439–45

Hume E (1990) The antisocial personality disorder diagnosis. *Am J Psychiatry* **147**: 1254

Luntz BK, Widom CS (1994) Antisocial personality disorder in abused and neglected children grown up. *Am J Psychiatry* **151**: 670–4

Mannuzza S, Klein RG, Bessler A, Malloy P, LaPadula M (1998) Adult psychiatric status of hyperactive boys grown up. *Am J Psychiatry* **155**: 493–8

Mathew RJ, Wilson WH, Blazer DG, George LK (1993) Psychiatric disorders in adult children of alcoholics: data from the Epidemiologic Catchment Area project. *Am J Psychiatry* **150**: 793–800

Myers MG, Stewart DG, Brown SA (1998) Progression from conduct disorder to antisocial personality disorder following treatment for adolescent substance abuse. *Am J Psychiatry* **155**: 479–85

North CS, Smith EM, Spitznagel EL (1993) Is antisocial personality a valid diagnosis among the homeless? *Am J Psychiatry* **150**: 578–83

Norton K, Hinshelwood RD (1996) Severe personality disorder. Treatment issues and selection for in-patient psychotherapy. *Br J Psychiatry* **168**: 723–31

Pfeffer CR, Plutchik R, Mizruchi MS (1983) Predictors of assaultiveness in latency age children. *Am J Psychiatry* **140**: 31–5

Pollock VE, Briere J, Schneider L, Knop J, Mednick SA, Goodwin DW (1990) Childhood antecedents of antisocial behavior: parental alcoholism and physical abusiveness. *Am J Psychiatry* **147**: 1290–3

Reich J, Thompson WD (1987) DSM-III Personality Disorder clusters in three populations. *Br J Psychiatry* **150**: 471

Reiss D, Hetherington EM, Plomin R *et al* (1995) Genetic questions for environmental studies. Differential parenting and psychopathology in adolescence. *Arch Gen Psychiatry* **52**: 925–36

Robins LN (1978) Sturdy childhood predictors of adult antisocial behaviour: replications from longitudinal studies. *Psychol Med* **8**: 611–22

Rounsaville BJ, Anton SF, Carroll K, Budde D, Prusoff BA, Gawin F (1991) Psychiatric diagnoses of treatment-seeking cocaine abusers. *Arch Gen Psychiatry* **48**: 43–51

Tantam D, Whittaker J (1992) Personality disorder and self-wounding. *Br J Psychiatry* **161**: 451

Thapar A, McGuffin P (1996) A twin study of antisocial and neurotic symptoms in childhood. *Psychol Med* **26**: 1111–8

Winston A, Laikin M, Pollack J, Samstag LW, McCullough L, Muran JC (1994) Short-term psychotherapy of personality disorders. *Am J Psychiatry* **151**: 190–4

10

Schizophrenia

History

- Previous diagnoses/episodes
  - ❑ personality disorder
  - ❑ affective disorder
  - ❑ drug-induced psychosis
  - ❑ other episode of strange or bizarre behaviour
- Gradual onset
- DSM-IV requires duration longer than 6 months
- Evidence of a precipitant
  - ❑ life event
- Symptomatology
  - ❑ first rank symptom in the absence of organic disease
  - ❑ catatonic symptoms
  - ❑ positive and negative symptoms
- Reason for coming to attention of the medical profession

Family history

- Evidence of a genetic component
  - ❑ schizophrenia
  - ❑ 'schizophrenia spectrum disorder'
- Evidence of high expressed emotion in the family
- Paternal occupation/social class (looking for evidence of social drift)

Personal history

- Season of birth
- Birth trauma
- Neurodevelopmental theory of schizophrenia
- Loner at school
- Being bullied, regarded as odd

- Migration
- Deterioration of personality
- Abrupt cessation of promising studies or career
- Difficulties at work
- Being sacked
- Finding it hard to concentrate/cope with the demands of work

Past medical history

- Diseases associated with psychosis
  - endocrine
    Cushing's disease, Addison's disease' Conn's disease
  - epilepsy
    temporal lobe epilepsy
  - head injury

Past psychiatric history

- Previous episodes/admissions to psychiatric hospital

Drug history

- Psychotropic drugs
  - neuroleptics, especially depot neuroleptic medication
- Prescribed drugs that can cause psychosis
  - anticholinergics
  - steroids

Pre-morbid personality

- Schizoid personality disorder
- Religious beliefs
  - need to establish presence of religious convictions that might render a potential delusion as culturally compatible
- Forensic history
  - previous convictions, with details of the offence and whether sentenced to hospital rather than prison
- Smoking
- Alcohol

❏ evidence of excessive use
- Illicit drugs
  - ❏ cocaine
  - ❏ amphetamines (including ecstasy and drugs for induction of weight loss)
  - ❏ cannabis
  - ❏ khat
  - ❏ benzodiazepine (regarding withdrawal)

Social circumstances

- Homelessness
- Unemployment
- Support by mental health services
  - ❏ community psychiatric nurse
  - ❏ psychiatric social worker
  - ❏ attendance at psychiatric day hospital or outpatient department
  - ❏ attendance at day centre
- Sickness benefit

Psychosexual history

- Lack of relationships

Mental state examination

Appearance

- Poor self care
- Clothing that might have special significance (in the context of a delusion)

Behaviour

- As though responding to hallucinations
- Carrying out a delusional task
- Appearing preoccupied with the internal world
- Adopting a strange posture
  - ❏ delusional
  - ❏ catatonia (eg, waxy flexibility)
- Bizarre gait
- Parkinsonian gait

- ❐ especially lack of arm swinging
- ◆ Evidence of side effects of neuroleptic medication
  - ❐ Parkinsonism — pill rolling tremor, hypersalivation, bizarre or rigid posture
  - ❐ dystonia, eg. torticollis
  - ❐ akathisia
  - ❐ oculogyric crisis
  - ❐ tardive dyskinesia, especially buccolinguomasticatory movements (the 'boiled sweet sign')
  - ❐ evidence of rabbit syndrome of Pisa syndrome

Mood

- ◆ May be euthymic, but may be elevated or depressed (anhedonia)

Affect

- ◆ Perplexed
- ◆ Incongruous
- ◆ Anxious
- ◆ Confused
- ◆ Child-like or giggly
- ◆ Mask-like
- ◆ Apathetic
- ◆ Blunted

Speech

- ◆ Evidence of thought disorder
  - ❐ word salad
  - ❐ knight's move thinking
  - ❐ derailment
  - ❐ neologisms

Thoughts

- ◆ Suicidal ideation
- ◆ Delusions
  - ❐ primary (autochthonous)
  - ❐ secondary

Experiences

- ◆ First rank symptoms
  - ❐ third person auditory hallucinations with running commentary

- ❑ passivity phenomena (made thoughts, actions, feelings)
- ❑ thought insertion, withdrawal, broadcasting; echo de la pensee, thought block
- ◆ Hallucinations
  - ❑ all modalities
  - ❑ functional, reflex, extracampine

Cognition

- ◆ Concrete thinking

Insight

- ◆ May be absent

Physical examination

- ◆ Soft neurological signs
- ◆ Motor disorder

Investigations

- ◆ Informant history
- ◆ Bloods to exclude a physical cause
- ◆ Urine drug screen
- ◆ CT scan, MRI scan
- ◆ PET scan
- ◆ EEG

Management

- ◆ Biological
  - ❑ neuroleptics (oral/depot)
- ◆ Psychological
  - ❑ family therapy
  - ❑ to reduce high expressed emotion
  - ❑ supportive therapy
  - ❑ visits from CPN
- ◆ Social
  - ❑ case management

- ❏ hospital admission
  inpatient / day patient
◆ Outpatient treatment
◆ Crisis intervention/early intervention service
◆ Occupational therapy
◆ Industrial therapy
◆ Sheltered workshop
◆ Day centre
◆ Housing
  - ❏ independent
  - ❏ landlady scheme
  - ❏ hostel
  - ❏ hospital hostel
◆ Financial support
◆ Support for patients, relatives and carers
  - ❏ National Schizophrenia Fellowship
  - ❏ MIND
  - ❏ SANE

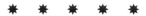

Schizophrenia is a complex disorder that, at present, has to be recognised on the basis of clinical symptoms. There is no diagnostic test and it is not clear whether what is lumped together under the rubric 'schizophrenia' represents one or several conditions. What is clear is that it represents a disturbance of individual mental functions, individually or in groups. The mental functions that are affected include thought process, perception, mood, belief and motivation. Abnormalities of thought, include:

- a jumbling of the thought processes — referred to as **formal thought disorder**. It is recognised by speech that does not make sense; for example, 'The type of apple that you when it is beyond the horizon can it take the basis of you know what I mean'
- a belief that the patient's thoughts are no longer private and can be heard by others — **thought broadcasting**
- that thoughts are being removed from the patient's head — **thought withdrawal**; or
- being placed in the patient's mind involuntarily — **thought insertion**.

Disorders of perception primarily include **hallucinations**. A hallucination is defined as a perception occurring in the absence of an external stimulus, ie. the person hears a voice although there is no one talking. It is important to remember that our perceptions are our realities and to the patient it is a real voice, not an imaginary one. It is, therefore, completely inappropriate to order a patient to believe that his experience is imaginary and to do so may be followed by a strong or even violent reaction — not completely inappropriate. However, it may be reasonable to explain to the patient that you recognise his experiences, but that they do not tally with yours. A tactful way of handling of the situation could be to agree that 'we beg to differ'. Hallucinations may occur in any sensory modality, but in schizophrenia the most common is to hear voices, feel unusual sensations in the body and experience strange smells, although visions and unusual taste sensations do occur.

Mood disturbances may include abnormal elation or depression, or perplexity associated with a feeling that something strange is happening, referred to as a **delusional mood**.

Abnormalities of belief are referred to as **delusions**, defined as a 'false, fixed belief that is not in keeping with the patient's social or cultural background.' Thus, a belief in the existence of God is not culturally abnormal, but the belief that I am the Son of God is. This is especially true when you disprove my belief logically by pointing out that my mother was not the Virgin Mary, a point with which I may concur.

Disorders of motivation may include a paralysing apathy in which even getting on with the basic chores of the day — getting up, washing, dressing — may be too much effort. Episodes such as this may occur acutely and resolve, or may persist over years, and it is often seen that over years there is a gradual decline of the personality.

For some patients, schizophrenia becomes a chronic condition. It is characterised by frequent relapses of acute symptoms against a background of gradual but definite deterioration. The patient treated for an acute episode may not quite get back to the level of functioning that he or she had before the episode.

As the patient recovers from an acute episode, there are several aspects of management that the doctor will need to consider. The first is to tell the patient and the relatives the diagnosis and discuss in general terms the long-term outlook. This may not be straightforward, as both the patient and the relative may be resistant to accepting the diagnosis, especially with its loss of aspirations for the future and social stigma. Even after acceptance, the diagnosis may not be fully understood and the doctor may need to spend some time explaining and supporting. The patient and family may wish for further details and the doctor should give information about self-help groups such as the National Schizophrenia Fellowship, MIND and SANE.

Aspects in the long-term management of the patient that need to be considered should include all aspects of the patient's life: accommodation, occupation, financial, relationships (especially with carers, such as other family members) and medical, in particular pharmacological. The support of social workers (including outreach workers) and paramedical staff (community psychiatric nurses, occupational therapists, clinical psychologists) may be enlisted to carry out many of these tasks. The doctor has the responsibility to ensure that arrangements are made for the patient to be reviewed regularly by him/herself or community psychiatric nurses.

When considering accommodation, the main concern is to ascertain the level of support the patient requires. Most patients and their relatives would prefer the patient to return home to parents or spouse. This is confirmed by Professor Eve Johnstone in her 10-year follow-up study of patients at Northwick Park Hospital. Care at home is not always possible and other options may need to be considered. For the most dependent patients, the support of a hostel, which looks like a hospital ward in a community setting ('hospital hostel') may be required. Those capable of a degree of self-care may be able to live in a residential hostel, where care staff are present, but expect residents to look after themselves. Some excellent hostels are provided by the social services. Charitable organisations also provide accommodation, such as the homes run by the Richmond Fellowship Foundation or the Carr-Gomm Society. Occasionally, mentally ill people who may have offended may be eligible for help from the National Association for the Care and Rehabilitation of Offenders (NACRO) who have some hostels. For those who are yet more independent, a group home, in which several discharged patients live together, with no care assistants on site, may be sufficient. Finally, there is independent living, although pressure on local borough councils is such that the demand for flats outstrips supply. This so acute that although people discharged from mental hospitals can be regarded as vulnerable people warranting priority in rehousing, there is rarely a flat available at the time a patient is ready to be discharged from hospital. Mentally ill people are often housed in unsatisfactory bed-and-breakfast accommodation, where the lack of cooking facilities and provided meals means that those with limited funds are forced to eat in restaurants or cafés, or buy takeaways; a costly way of eating. It is not surprising that such patients often relapse and have to return to hospital. This happens so frequently that it has been referred to as the **revolving door syndrome**. Others, for whom the situation breaks down completely, can be found living on the streets. This may become a way of life, perhaps interspersed with brief periods of living in a hostel for the homeless. The situation is sufficiently frequent for Inner London councils to employ psychiatrists and general practitioners to treat this group of people.

The occupation of the discharged patient depends on the effects of the illness on his/her intellectual capacity and ability to function within the bounds of society. Many patients can work without their employers or colleagues being made aware of their illness. Some employers are very supportive and understanding when informed of the patient's illness. In the author's experience, organisations, such as Waitrose, Camden Council, British Telecom and the former British Rail, have been willing to accept employees' need to take time off during periods of illness and hold open positions until patients can return to their post. In the UK, companies have a statutory duty to ensure that 3% of those they employ come from the ranks of the disabled, and a patient with chronic schizophrenia would fall into this category. Such patients may have no difficulty carrying out a manual job (filling shelves, gardening, etc) and patients who are capable may carry out more complex clerical tasks.

However, if such work is not available, or if the patient's motivation is so impaired that he is viewed as unreliable by an employer, sheltered occupation may be of benefit. Some units are based around industrial therapy units of mental hospitals, but these are disappearing as mental hospitals close. Separate initiatives have been developed in the community, but their provision is still inadequate. Other provision includes local authority day centres, where patients are occupied rather than employed. Some patients use the time for retraining and there are several adult education courses that can be helpful.

For those in employment, the financial problems are the same as for those without mental illness. There is a range of benefits to which the unemployed may be entitled, although the amounts are small. Help from a social worker may be essential, if patients are to obtain such benefits and then manage to budget the limited amount received. An additional problem, for those receiving benefits prior to admission, is that such benefits can be reduced, after six weeks in hospital, to a few pounds a week, ie, pocket money. Return to higher levels of benefit is permitted on discharge, but for some the bureaucratic process may be so slow that it may be several weeks before patients receive money to which they are entitled. This causes additional hardship.

Much research has been conducted to uncover the factors in the home and family environment that contribute to the causation of schizophrenia. In the 1950s, the concept of the 'schizophrenogenic mother' was generated, an explanation that has no basis in fact. Attaching blame to a heavily involved carer at a time when she is greatly distressed by the realisation of the terrible affliction that has affected her child, is to say the least, unkind. Another theory was that of 'double-bind' communication (Bateson *et al*, 1956). This suggested that parents of such children were giving one communication verbally and its exact opposite non-verbally; for example, telling a child he can invite a friend to tea and treating it as a terrible crime when he does. Schizophrenia was postulated as a solution to this insoluble problem. Such an explanation has not been helpful.

However, the theory of **expressed emotion** has proved useful, especially combined with the view that schizophrenia is basically a disease with a biological origin. The theory is that, in families who communicate with high expressed emotion, a patient with schizophrenia is more likely to become ill than in a family with low expressed emotion. The term 'expressed emotion' is understood to mean a situation in which a person frequently expresses his/her emotions about another person, eg. by shouting at them and making hostile comments. The advantage of this theory is that it can be used in a non-blaming manner. It allows for the possibility that this way of communicating may have arisen in a family as an understandable response to the development of schizophrenia. In his/her early and unrecognised stages, the schizophrenic is often perceived by the family as lazy, lacking interest in the family and not pulling his/her weight. This theory can help the family not only to cope, but do something positive to help the situation. The treatment is referred to as family therapy for expressed emotions, and is more directive and specific than the meaning of family therapy in psychotherapy.

Neuroleptic medication, when shown to be effective, has been used in the treatment of the acutely ill patient where it can bring about a resolution of symptoms, and to prevent or reduce the number of subsequent relapses (**maintenance therapy**). The doctor often has problems ensuring that patients take medication, that their condition is regularly monitored to ensure continued good health without undue side-effects and to detect relapse early. The medication can be prescribed as an oral preparation, to be taken one or more times a day, and the patient can be seen in the outpatient department. However, even well-intentioned patients find this is a difficult regime and may fail to comply. Pills may be missed and patients may fail to attend the outpatient clinic. Thus, the doctor may have to make sporadic assessments in the artificial environment of the clinic about how much medication has been actually taken and how the patient has been coping. Alternatively, neuroleptic medication can be given in an oily vehicle by injection into a muscle, from where the drug can leak out slowly into the bloodstream. This can be effective if given at intervals of between one and four weeks. A community psychiatric nurse, who can also take the opportunity to assess the patient, often in his/her own home, can give the injection. The nurse can remind the patient of outpatient appointments and give collateral information to the doctor about the mental health of the patient between appointments, allowing for a much more satisfactory assessment of the efficacy of treatment.

History of presenting complaint

Over the last century, there has been much discussion about the nature of schizophrenia, its symptomatology and natural history. The tradition in Europe has followed the suggestion of Schneider (1959) that there are a number of symptoms, which, in the absence of organic disease, should be considered in the first rank for a diagnosis of schizophrenia. The scientific validity of 'first-rank symptoms' has been questioned (Crichton, 1996), but they remain in widespread clinical use. The distinction between positive and negative symptoms of schizophrenia, which have been observed clinically, has been supported by CT findings and has prognostic value (Andreasen and Olsen, 1982; Eaton *et al*, 1995; Hwu *et al*, 1995). More recently, different syndromes (psychomotor poverty, disorganisation and reality distortion) have been identified on the basis of neuroimaging studies (Liddle *et al*, 1992), but these have not yet been integrated into clinical practice or the major diagnostic classifications.

The course of schizophrenia varies. Some patients recover from the initial episode without further recurrence, but many have further episodes. Of these, psychosis may resolve completely or partially for varying periods of time. Life events can precipitate acute episodes of schizophrenia (Birley and Brown, 1970, Norman and Malla, 1993a and 1993b). Following admission to hospital, symptoms improve over the first six months, but those symptoms left at 12 months are likely to be present at 24 months (Wittenborn, 1977)

Family history

There is evidence to support a genetic component to schizophrenia. Compared to an incidence in the population of 1%, Zerbin-Rudin (1967) found an incidence of 4% in parents of patients with schizophrenia; 8% in siblings and 12% in children. Essen-Moller (1963) found a ratio between monozygotic and dizygotic twins for incidence of schizophrenia of 69:13. Even after applying DSM-III diagnoses to the early twin series of Gottesman and Shields, heritability was still found to be 0.85% for schizophrenia (Farmer *et al*, 1987). In the adopted children of parents with schizophrenia, both Heston (1966) and Rosenthal (1971) found an increased rate among adopted away offspring of index patients. Bassett *et al* (1988) described a case of a patient and uncle with distinctive facial dysmorphism and schizophrenia associated with a translocation on chromosome 5, leading to investigation of family pedigrees and evidence supportive of Bassett's findings by Sherrington (1988), but not by Kennedy (1988). An editorial in the *Lancet* (1989) discusses this early research into the genetics of schizophrenia. More recent research has focussed on the molecular biology, with evidence for linkage at the 6p, 8p (Kendler *et al*, 1996) and 22q loci (Kennedy, 1996).

Family studies have, at times, suggested that schizophrenia is part of a 'spectrum of clinical syndromes that includes schizoaffective disorder, other nonaffective psychoses, schizotypal personality disorder, and probably psychotic affective illness, but not nonpsychotic affective illness' (Kendler *et al*, 1995) or anxiety disorders (Kendler and Gardner, 1997). Vaughn and Leff (1976) have indicated how the presence of high expressed emotion in the family might contribute to the aggravation of psychosis in a patient with schizophrenia. Kavanagh (1992) provides a review of the area. There is evidence for some stability of expressed emotion over time, associated with a higher rate of relapse, but even in high expressed emotion situations, there are episodes of relapse when expressed emotion is low. Thus the relationship between high expressed emotion and relapse is more complex than was originally thought (McCreadie *et al*, 1993). Recent research shows that high expressed emotion is associated with sustained distress in the relatives and a longer caring history (Barrowclough and Parle, 1997).

It is also useful to know the place of residence and occupation of parents and siblings of a patient, as they may show a contrast that will suggest social drift. In this phenomenon, patients from well-to-do backgrounds slip down the social scale as a result of their illness.

Personal history

Recently, it has been recognised that schizophrenia may be a disorder involving faulty development. Subtle brain damage *in utero* in perinatal development, or in early childhood, if occurring in brain systems that do not become active until after puberty, may be the basis of a disorder that does not manifest itself until late adolescence or early adulthood. This is known as the neurodevelopmental theory of schizophrenia (Waddington, 1993). Maternal influenza in the second trimester may be associated with schizophrenia (Adams *et al*, 1993; Wright *et al*, 1995). Crow and Done (1992) do not agree. Small head circumference at birth, suggestive of genetic or intrauterine antepartum problems, is more common in patients with schizophrenia (Hultman *et al*,1997). Obstetric complications, such as abnormal presentations at birth and complicated Caesarian births are found more frequently in patients with early onset schizophrenia (Verdoux *et al*,1997). There is longitudinal prospective evidence that patients with high biological risk who develop schizophrenia spectrum disorder were 'passive babies who exhibited short attention spans. In school, they experienced interpersonal difficulties and displayed disturbing behaviour, reflecting poor affective control. Examination of childhood home movies of patients with a diagnosis of schizophrenia suggests that pre-schizophrenic females show less expressions of joy and pre-schizophrenic children of both sexes display a greater proportion of negative affect than their normal siblings (Walker *et al*, 1993). From clinical assessments at a mean of 15 years of age, formal cognitive disturbance and defective emotional rapport emerged as pre-morbid characteristics' (Parnas *et al*, 1982). In childhood, patients who subsequently develop schizophrenia often give a history of isolating themselves from their peers at school and, on occasions, being the victim of bullying. There is some evidence that patients who develop schizophrenia have histories of poor sociability in childhood and adolescence, and impaired school adjustment (Cannon *et al*, 1997). Even this theory is subject to constant revision of the data, and with the findings of similarities between childhood and adult types of schizophrenia, the exact nature of the neuroplasticity is being questioned (Nasrallah and Tolbert, 1997).

Schizophrenia does not always manifest itself in early adolescence. The peak ages of onset are 18–25 years for men and 23–35 years for women, and the age range for first diagnosis in one study was 12–78 years, with approximately 30% first being diagnosed after the age of 30 years (Gorwood *et al*, 1995). Thus, many people who develop the disease manage to start a working life before becoming ill. Complaints, such as difficulties at work, failing to cope with work and being sacked, are not in any way specific to schizophrenia. However, in a patient who presents with these and other symptoms of schizophrenia, it may indicate a more slow and insidious onset than the presentation initially suggested, and have prognostic significance.

In the long-term course of schizophrenia, a typical clinical observation is that there is intellectual decline. In view of the more recent pre-morbid findings, this has been questioned. There is some evidence that in patients destined to develop chronic schizophrenia in adulthood, deficits in IQ were present in childhood and were stable 20 years later, ie. in the early stage of the disease (Russell *et al*, 1997).

Past medical history

A fuller definition of 'first rank symptoms' is that these symptoms are in the first rank of symptoms for the diagnosis of schizophrenia in the absence of organic pathology. The clinical picture of first rank symptoms seems to be the picture observed when the brain has undergone certain types of insult, of which schizophrenia is only one. The purpose of considering the past medical history of a patient when a diagnosis of schizophrenia is being considered is to make a differential diagnosis with medical illnesses whose treatment might resolve the clinical picture. There has been recognition for many years that certain endocrine syndromes can present with a psychosis, ie. Cushing's disease, Addison's or Conn's; the cost of a routine blood tests such as urea and electrolytes is sufficiently small to warrant exclusion. The clinician should be clear that in UK practice, such results in a population of psychiatric inpatients only rarely reveal an underlying medical condition and some have advocated a white cell count and thyroid function tests as the only cost-effective investigations (White and Barraclough, 1989). The relationship between schizophrenia and epilepsy has been much debated (Mace, 1993; Fiordelli *et al*, 1993). Syndromes such as head injury, puerperal psychosis and delirium tremens in alcohol withdrawal can present as a schizophreniform psychosis.

It is also important to consider the presence or history of medical conditions whose treatment may cause psychosis as a side-effect (eg. asthma treated by corticosteroids, recent operation followed by a post-operative psychosis). However, in around 5% of first episode presentations, there will be an organic cause (Johnstone *et al*,1987), such as syphilis, sarcoidosis, carcinoma of lung, autoimmune multisystem disease, cerebral cysticercosis, thyroid disease and previous head injury.

Past psychiatric history

As schizophrenia is a chronic relapsing and remitting illness, previous episodes may have occurred. As with all previous episodes, case notes should be sought, and hospitals, doctors and treatment centres should be recorded carefully. This is less important in the examination, but relevant to clinical practice. A feature, which distinguishes between the chronic course of bipolar affective illness and schizophrenia, is that, in affective disorder, the person may function normally at times of remission. In schizophrenia there is a gradual decline, accompanied by a failure to return completely to the previous level of functioning after each new episode of acute psychosis. This distinction is often blurred in clinical practice, but should be sought.

First rank symptoms do occur in other psychiatric syndromes and this should be considered in the differential diagnosis. Hypomania (Brockington *et al*, 1980), puerperal psychosis (Dean and Kendell, 1981; Harding, 1989), delirium tremens (Kramp *et al*, 1979) and head injury should all be considered in the differential diagnosis.

Drug history

A history of neuroleptic medication, especially in depot form, is strongly suggestive that a diagnosis of schizophrenia has been previously made. Potentially, any medication can affect the brain and cause an organic syndrome that presents as a schizophreniform psychosis. Certain drugs are known to have an increased risk, for example, dopamine agonists, such as bromocriptine; steroids (Hall *et al*, 1979) and anticholinergic drugs. There have been reports of psychoses following ceftazidine (Al-Zahawi *et al*, 1988), salbutamol (Khanna and Davies, 1986), quinidine (Deleu and Schmedding, 1987), fenfluramine (Murphy and Watters, 1986) and abuse of Actifed (Leighton, 1982).

Pre-morbid personality

Part of early clinical descriptions of schizophrenia included the term 'deterioration of the personality'. To demonstrate this, it is necessary to know what the personality was before deterioration. For example, a hard-working and well-motivated person who becomes severely apathetic; or a person who has always paid attention to his/her grooming, but presents with poor self-care represents a change that may be a deterioration of personal behaviour.

The nature of pre-morbid personality traits in schizophrenia is complex. Recent work suggests that explosive, paranoid and schizoid personality traits (not necessarily in the same individuals) are more commonly found to precede schizophrenia than other non-organic psychoses (Dalkin *et al*, 1994). The majority of patients who develop schizophrenia do not commit homicide. The rate of homicide committed by mentally abnormal offenders does not seem to vary with the overall rate of homicide in a community (Coid, 1983).

Drug use

Frequently, patients with schizophrenia smoke cigarettes and prevalence in one series of outpatients was estimated at 88% (Hughes *et al*, 1986). There is some evidence that patients with co-morbid substance abuse and schizophrenia had better pre-morbid adjustment, suggesting the possibility of a two-stage model in which increased sociability increases exposure to opportunities of substance use in a subset of patients. Subsequent onset of psychotic illness accelerates the use to a pathological level as the individual attempts to cope with the stress of the developing mental illness. (Arndt *et al*, 1992).

Many people in the general population take psychoactive drugs that can cause psychoses. In particular, up to 4% take cannabis and around 1% stimulants, such as amphetamines, on a regular basis (Ramsay and Percy, 1996). Chronic excessive alcohol intake can also cause a hallucinosis. Withdrawal from alcohol or benzodiazepines in a patient dependent on either or both of these drugs can manifest as a psychosis. Thus, these drugs should always be sought in patients who present as psychotic. Among known psychiatric patients, the incidence of psychoactive drug use is high. The odds ratio for a patient with a mental disorder also having a drug misuse disorder was 2:3 in the Epidemiological Catchment Area study, Regier *et al*, 1990). This can precipitate a new episode of psychosis or retard recovery from an acute episode. Whether cannabis causes schizophrenia remains controversial, but there is some evidence to suggest this may be so from a long-term follow-up study of conscripts (Andréasson *et al*, 1987). The evidence is questioned in Thomas (1993) and has been challenged by a study of the recent rise in teenage cannabis use in Australia. This has not shown an accompanying rise in incidence of schizophrenia (Hall and Solowij, 1997).

It seems that psychoactive drug-taking is a serious problem for patients with established schizophrenia. Poor compliance with medication, alcohol and psychoactive drug use are factors that are associated with numbers of readmissions to hospital (Sullivan *et al*, 1995; Haywood *et al*, 1995).

Intelligence

There is evidence that low IQ is a risk factor for subsequent development of schizophrenia (David *et al*, 1997).

Social circumstances

A number of people who have schizophrenia lose their accommodation, although the relationship between mental illness and homelessness is not simple (Scott, 1993). There is an increased prevalence in cities compared to rural areas, explained by a social drift of mentally ill people to inner cities. This has been questioned and it has been proposed that an environmental factor in cities may be aetiological in the development of schizophrenia (Lewis *et al*, 1992).

Antisocial personality disorder and substance abuse are widespread among indigent patients with schizophrenia, who are either homeless or in a mental health programme. Such patients have been found to have more disrupted early lives and to greater problems with drug use, but no differences in key aspects of schizophrenia. (Caton *et al*, 1994).

Psychosexual history

There is evidence suggesting patients with schizophrenia reproduce at a rate about a quarter that of normal controls (Kendler *et al*, 1995).

Mental state examination

This is well-covered in standard textbooks, usually in descriptive format. A few recent points are noted here. Recent studies have provided support for the clinical impression that affective flattening does seem to occur in patients with chronic schizophrenia, but not in patients with mania (Reddy *et al*, 1992). Studies of the speech of patients with schizophrenia suggest that it is syntactically less complex than controls (Thomas *et al*, 1996). This appears to be a component of the acute illness and not a pre-morbid trait (Done *et al*, 1998). Features of difficulties in the sentence structure of patients include vague references, confused references, missing information, ambiguous word meanings, wrong word references and lack of structural clarity (Docherty *et al*, 1996). These describe the abnormalities of speech experienced by the examiner as formal thought disorder ('word salad'). Evidence suggests that the complexity and integrity of speech deteriorate over time (King *et al*, 1990).

In respect of somatic delusions, there is a difference between parts of the body to which disorder is ascribed and laterality. Patients with schizophrenia localise on the left and those with affective disorder on the right (McGilchrist and Cutting, 1995). It would appear that there are subtle cognitive deficits in schizophrenia, such as difficulties in problem solving and visual memory (Goldberg *et al*, 1993). There is evidence that reading and spelling ability are maintained even when IQ is lowered in schizophrenia and mania, giving a useful indication of pre-morbid intelligence (Dalby and Williams, 1986). However, the suggestion that patients with schizophrenia are prone to concrete thinking has been questioned (Cutting and Ryan, 1982), with the suggestion that patients have an abnormal way of categorising the world.

Physical examination

Minor neurological abnormalities are found more frequently in patients with schizophrenia and their relatives than in patients with affective disorder and substance misuse or normal controls (Kinney *et al*, 1986).

Investigations

Blood tests

It has been questioned whether there is any benefit in carrying out more than estimation of white blood cell count and thyroid function, and perhaps syphilis serology, in patients who do not show clinical signs of physical illness (White and Barraclough, 1989).

Radiology

There is evidence that chest X-ray of a patient with schizophrenia or other functional psychosis in general adult patients is unlikely to reveal any abnormality in the absence of chest symptoms (Hughes and Barraclough, 1980). Similarly, skull X-ray is unlikely to be helpful routinely (White and Barraclough, 1986).

EEG

EEG is not carried out as a routine clinical procedure. Differences between patients with schizophrenia and controls have been observed (Shagass, 1982), but it does not appear that such differences are diagnostic.

Management

Schizophrenia has been increasingly recognised by medical practitioners over the past 100 years, and there have been a variety of treatments: biological, psychological and social. Some treatments, such as insulin coma therapy or dynamic psychotherapy, have been abandoned as ineffective or even harmful. Nevertheless, all three modalities have a part to play in treating and ameliorating the disabilities of the chronically impaired patient.

Pharmacological

Neuroleptic medication has been the mainstay of drug treatment since its discovery in the 1950s. It has been established that this is not a placebo effect (Johnstone *et al*, 1978). A 150mg dose of chlorpromazine daily has been identified as the minimum required to exert an antipsychotic effect that is better than placebo. The effect is dose-related, such that a dose of 300mg and 400 mg daily give an improved response (Curry, 1986). Evidence shows that there is little extra antipsychotic effect at a dose above 600mg chlorpromazine daily (Baldessarini *et al*, 1988) or flupenthixol decanoate 40mg fortnightly (McCreadie *et al*, 1979).

Original neuroleptics were thought to be effective against positive symptoms of schizophrenia, but less so against negative symptoms. The focus of research was on the dopamine receptor. This was based on the dopamine hypothesis of schizophrenia. For the first generation of antipsychotics, typical daily doses of antipsychotic correlated well with binding to dopamine receptors (Seeman *et al*, 1976), especially the dopamine D2 receptor — one of at least five subclasses. Further research has focussed on treatment of negative symptoms. Following successful treatment of patients, who had previously been neuroleptic refractory, with clozapine, whose binding to the D2 receptor is very limited, and with risperidone, where there is significant activity at the 5HT2 receptor, it is now clear that several receptors are involved in the schizophrenic psychosis. Other neurotransmitters systems that have been implicated include glutamate, cholecystokinin and possibly opiates (Pickar, 1995; Sedvall and Farde, 1995). As well as targeting different receptors, psychopharmacology development has involved selecting out dopamine receptor subtypes in an effort to reduce the incidence of extrapyramidal side-effects.

Prescribers should be aware of the complications of neuroleptic therapy, which are many, and their management. Of particular importance are extrapyramidal side-effects and their treatment with anticholinergic medication, (WHO, 1990), akathisia (Halstead *et al*, 1994), dystonia (Owens, 1990), tardive dyskinesia (Bergen *et al*, 1989) and neuroleptic malignant syndrome (Kellam, 1990).

Psychological

Individual treatment

In the management of chronically ill patients with schizophrenia, the situation can be alleviated by shaping the patient's behaviour and improving practical function. One method to do this is by using a token economy (Fullerton et al, 1978; Scott and Wood, 1987). In patients whose auditory hallucinations do not respond sufficiently to neuroleptic treatment, audiotape therapy has been tried (McInnis and Marks, 1990; Nelson et al, 1991). So, too, have earplugs and subvocal counting (Nelson et al, 1991). More recently, techniques of cognitive behavioural therapy for patients with chronic schizophrenia have been developed that seem to produce improvements in symptoms and reduce relapse rates (Tarrier et al, 1998).

Family treatment

In line with the theory of expressed emotion, a specific form of family therapy has been suggested in which an attempt is made to reduce the expressed emotion in communication within the family. There is some evidence that this approach is helpful (Leff et al, 1990).

Social

In the treatment of acutely ill patients with schizophrenia, while many will require inpatient admission, a small proportion can be acutely admitted to a day hospital (Creed *et al*, 1990). After discharge, a number of patients will have chronic disorders and will need continuing support. Placing patients who need a high level of continuing support in community hostel wards has had some degree of success (Creighton *et al*, 1991). For patients who can live more independently, attendance at a day centre may be helpful (Lancet, 1985). Patients living independently are often in contact with mental health professionals (Melzer *et al*, 1991), such as a community psychiatric nurse (CPN). CPNs often concentrate on administration of medication and practical help with social problems, such as housing or benefits (Muijen *et al*, 1994). Social support through a network service may be helpful: for a group of chronic patients such a service did not affect symptoms, but did improve social functioning in respect of slowness, personal hygiene and posturing (Thornicroft and Breakey, 1991).

In considering placement, it is more likely that it is the quality of the environment, not its situation in hospital or the community that is responsible for improvements in the functioning of chronically ill patients (Rodriguez-Ferrera and Vassilas, 1998).

Treatment for the family

It is distressing to have a mentally ill family member, but a proportion of carers do so without experiencing psychological distress. Distress in carers seems to be greater when the patient is passive in his use of time, ie. watching TV, listening to music, or sleeping (Oldridge and Hughes, 1992). Parents whose children develop schizophrenia develop a grief reaction that is chronic. It would seem that such parents have a reduced divorce rate (12% compared with 56% national average in the US). Unlike parents who lose a child through head injury or death, whose grief is intense acutely but eases over time, parents of a patient with chronic schizophrenia grieve much less at the time of diagnosis, but have exacerbation of grief feeling when the patient has an acute relapse. (Atkinson, 1994).

References

Adams W, Kendell RE, Hare EH, Munk-Jørgensen P (1993) Epidemiological evidence that maternal influenza contributes to the aetiology of schizophrenia. An analysis of Scottish, English and Danish data. *Br J Psychiatry* 163: 522–34

Al-Zahawi MF,Sprott MS, Hendrick DJ (1988) Hallucinations in association with ceftazidime. *Br Med J* **297**: 858

Andreasen N, Olsen S (1982) Negative *v* positive schizophrenia. Definition and validation. *Arch Gen Psychiatry* **39**: 789–94

Andréasson S, Allebeck P, Engström A, Rydberg U (1987) Cannabis and schizophrenia: a longitudinal study of Swedish conscripts. *Lancet* **ii**: 1483–86

Anon (1985) Day Hospitals for psychiatric care. *Lancet* **ii**: 1106–7

Anon (1989) Genetics of schizophrenia. *Lancet* **i**: 79–80

Arndt S, Tyrrell G, Flaum M, Andreasen NC (1992) Comorbidity of substance abuse and schizophrenia: the role of pre-morbid adjustment. *Psychol Med* **22**: 379–88

Atkinson SD (1994) Grieving and loss in parents with a schizophrenic child. *Am J Psychiatry* **151**: 1137–9

Baldessarini RJ, Cohen BM, Teichner MH (1988) Significance of neuroleptic dose and plasma level in the pharmacological treatment of psychoses. *Arch Gen Psychiatry* **45**: 79–91

Barrowclough C, Parle M (1997) Appraisal, psychological adjustment and expressed emotion in relatives of patients suffering from schizophrenia. *Br J Psychiatry* **171**: 26–30

Bassett AS, McGillivray BC, Jones BD, Pantzar JT (1988) Partial trisomy chromosome 5 cosegregating with schizophrenia. *Lancet* **i**: 799–801

Bateson G, Jackson DD, Haley J and Weakland JH (1956) Toward a theory of schizophrenia. *Behavioral Science* 1:251–64

Bergen JA, Eyland EA, Campbell *et al* (1989) The course of tardive dyskinesia in patients on long-term neuroleptics. *Br J Psychiatry* **154**: 523

Birley JLT, Brown GW (1970) Crisis and life changes preceding the onset or relapse of acute schizophrenia: clinical aspects. *Br J Psychiatry* **116**: 327–33

Brockington IF, Wainwright S, Kendall RE (1980) Manic patients with schizophrenic or paranoid symptoms. *Psychol Med* **10**: 73–83

Cannon M, Jones P, Gilvarry C, *et al* (1997) pre-morbid social functioning in schizophrenia and bipolar disorder: similarities and differences. *Am J Psychiatry* **154**: 1544–50

Caton CL, Shrout PE, Eagle PF, Opler LA, Felix A (1994) Correlates of codisorders in homeless and never homeless indigent schizophrenic men. *Psychol Med* **24**: 681–8

Coid J (1983) The epidemiology of abnormal homicide and murder followed by suicide. *Psychol Med* **13**: 855–60

Creed F, Black D, Anthony P, Osborn M, Thomas P, Tomenson B (1990) Randomised controlled trial of day patient versus inpatient psychiatric treatment. *Br Med J* **300**: 1033–7

Creighton FJ, Hyde CE, Farragher B (1991) Douglas House. Seven years' experience of a community hostel ward. *Br J Psychiatry* **159**: 500–4

Crichton P (1996) First rank symptoms or rank-and-file symptoms? *Br J Psychiatry* **169**: 537–50

Schizophrenia

Crow TJ, Done DJ (1992) Prenatal exposure to influenza does not cause schizophrenia. *Br J Psychiatry* **161**: 390–3

Curry SH (1986) Applied clinical pharmacology of schizophrenia. In: Bradley PB, Hirsch SR, eds. *The Psychopharmacology and Treatment of Schizophrenia*. Oxford University Press, Oxford

Cutting J, Ryan K (1982) The appreciation of imagery by schizophrenics: an interpretation of Goldstein's impairment of the abstract attitude. *Psychol Med* **12**: 585–90

Dalby JT, Williams R (1986) Preserved reading and spelling ability in psychotic disorders. *Psychol Med* **16**: 171–5

Dalkin T, Murphy P, Glazebrook C, Medley I, Harrison G (1994) pre-morbid personality in first-onset psychosis. *Br J Psychiatry* **164**: 202–7

David AS, Malmberg A, Brandt L, Allebeck P, Lewis G (1997) IQ and risk for schizophrenia: a population-based cohort study. *Psychol Med* **27**: 1311–23

Dean C, Kendell RE (1981) The symptomatology of puerperal illnesses. *Br J Psychiatry* **139**: 128–33

Deleu D, Schmedding E (1987) Acute psychosis as idiosyncratic reaction to quinidine: report of 2 cases. *Br Med J* **294**: 1001–2

Docherty NM, DeRosa M, Andreasen NC (1996) Communication disturbances in schizophrenia and mania. *Arch Gen Psychiatry* **53**: 358–64

Done DJ, Leinoneen E, Crow TJ, Sacker A (1998) Linguistic performance in children who develop schizophrenia in adult life. Evidence for normal syntactic ability. *Br J Psychiatry* **172**: 130–5

Eaton WW, Thara R, Federman B, Melton B, Liang K-Y (1995) Structure and course of positive and negative symptoms in schizophrenia. *Arch Gen Psychiatry* **52**: 127–34

Farmer AE, McGuffin P, Gottesman II (1987) Twin concordance for DSM-III schizophrenia. Scrutinizing the validity of the definition. *Arch Gen Psychiatry* **44**: 634–41

Fiordelli E, Beghi E, Bogliun G, Crespi V (1993) Epilepsy and psychiatric disturbance. A cross sectional study. *Br J Psychiatry* **163**: 446–50

Fullerton DT, Cayner JJ, McLaughlin-Reidel T (1978) Results of a token economy. *Arch Gen Psychiatry* **35**: 1451–3

Goldberg TE, Gold JM, Greenberg R *et al* (1993) Contrasts between patients with affective disorders and patients with schizophrenia on a neuropsychological test battery. *Am J Psychiatry* **150**: 1355–62

Gorwood P, Leboyer M, Jay M, Payan C, Feingold J (1995) Gender and age at onset in schizophrenia: impact of family history. *Am J Psychiatry* **152**: 208–12

Hall RCW, Popkin MK, Stickney SK, Gardner ER (1979) Presentation of the steroid psychoses. *J Nerv Ment Dis* **167**: 229–36

Hall W, Solowij N (1997) Long-term cannabis use and mental health. *Br J Psychiatry* **171**: 107

Halstead SM, Barnes TRE, Speller JC (1994) Akathisia: prevalence and associated dysphoria in an in-patient population with chronic schizophrenia. *Br J Psychiatry* **164**: 177

Harding JJ (1989) Postpartum psychiatric disorders: a review. *Comprehen Psychiatry* **30**: 109–12

Haywood TW, Kravitz HM, Grossman LS, Cavanaugh Jr, JL, Davis JM, Lewis DA (1995) Predicting the "revolving door" phenomenon among patients with schizophrenic, schizoaffective, and affective disorders. *Am J Psychiatry* **152**: 856–61

Heston LL (1966) Psychiatric disorders in foster home reared children of schizophrenic mothers. *Br J Psychiatry* **112**: 819–25

Hughes J, Barraclough BM (1980) Value of routine chest radiography in psychiatric patients. *Br Med J* **281**: 1461–2

Hughes JR, Hatsukami DK, Mitchell JE, Dahlgren LA (1986) Prevalence of smoking among psychiatric outpatients. *Am J Psychiatry* **143**: 993–7

Hwu H-G, Tan H, Chen C-C, Yeh L-L (1995) Negative symptoms at discharge predict poor outcome in schizophrenia. *Br J Psychiatry* **166**: 61–7

Hultman CM, Öhman A, Cnattingius S, Wieselgren I-M, Lindström LH (1997) Prenatal and neonatal risk factors for schizophrenia. *Br J Psychiatry* **170**: 128–33

Johnstone EC *et al* (1978) Mechanism of the antipsychotic effect in the treatment of acute schizophrenia. *Lancet* **ii**: 848–57

Johnstone EC, Macmillan JF, Crow TJ (1987) The occurrence of organic disease of possible or probable aetiological significance in a population of 268 cases of first episode schizophrenia. *Psychol Med* **17**: 371–9

Kavanagh DJ (1992) Recent developments in expressed emotion and schizophrenia. *Br J Psychiatry* **160**: 601–20

Kellam AMP (1990) The (frequently) neuroleptic (potentially) malignant syndrome. *Br J Psychiatry* **157**: 169

Kendler KS, McGuire M, Gruenberg AM, O'Hare A, Spellman M, Walsh D (1993) The Roscommon Family Study. I. Methods, diagnosis of probands, and risk of schizophrenia in relatives. *Arch Gen Psychiatry* **50**: 527–40

Kendler KS, MacLean CJ, O'Neill FA *et al* (1996) Evidence for a Schizophrenia Vulnerability Locus on Chromosome 8p in the Irish Study of High-Density Schizophrenia Families. *Am J Psychiatry* **153**: 1534–40

Kendler KS, Gardner CO (1997) The risk for psychiatric disorders in relatives of schizophrenic and control probands: a comparison of three independent studies. *Psychol Med* **27**: 411–9

Kennedy JL, Giuffra LA, Moises HW *et al* (1988) Evidence against linkage of schizophrenia to markers on chromosome 5 in a northern Swedish pedigree. *Nature* **336**: 167–70

Kennedy JL (1996) Schizophrenia genetics: the quest for an anchor. *Am J Psychiatry* **153**: 1513–4

Khanna PB, Davies R (1986) Hallucinations associated with the administration of salbutamol via a nebuliser. *Br Med J* **292**: 1430

King K, Fraser WI, Thomas P, Kendell RE (1990) Re-examination of the language of psychotic subjects. *Br J Psychiatry* **156**: 211–15

Kinney DK, Woods BT, Yurgelun-Todd D (1986) Neurologic abnormalities in schizophrenic patients and their families. II. Neurologic and psychiatric findings in relatives. *Arch Gen Psychiatry* **43**: 665–8

Kramp P, Hemingsen R (1979) Delirium tremens. Some clinical features. Part I. *Acta Psychiatr Scand* **60**: 393–404

Kramp P, Hemingsen R, Rafaelsen OJ (1979) Delirium tremens. Some clinical features. Part II. *Acta Psychaitr Scand* **60**: 405–22

Leff J, Berkowitz R, Shavit N, Strachan A, Glass I, Vaughn C (1990) A trial of family therapy v. a relatives group for schizophrenia. Two year follow-up. *Br J Psychiatry* **157**: 571

Leighton KM (1982) Paranoid psychosis after abuse of Actifed. *Br Med J* **284**: 789–90

Lewis G, David A, Andréasson S, Allebeck P (1992) Schizophrenia and city life. *Lancet* **340**: 137–40

Liddle PF, Friston KJ, Frith CD, Hirsch SR, Jones T, Frackowiak RSJ (1992) Patterns of cerebral blood flow in schizophrenia. *Br J Psychiatry* **160**: 179–86

Mace CJ (1993) Epilepsy and schizophrenia. *Br J Psychiatry* **163**: 439–45

McCreadie RG, Flanagan WL, McKnight J, Jorgensen A (1979) High dose flupenthixol decanoate in chronic schizophrenia. *Br J Psychiatry* **135**: 175–9

McCreadie RG, Robertson LJ, Hall DJ, Berry I (1993) The Nithsdale Schizophrenia Surveys. XI: Relatives' expressed emotion. Stability over five years and its relation to relapse. *Br J Psychiatry* **162**: 393–7

McGilchrist I, Cutting J (1995) Somatic delusions in schizophrenia and the affective psychoses. *Br J Psychiatry* **167**: 350–61

McInnis M, Marks I (1990) Audiotape therapy for persistent auditory hallucinations. *Br J Psychiatry* **157**: 913

Melzer D, Hale AS, Malik SJ, Hogman GA, Wood S (1991) Community care for patients with schizophrenia one year after hospital discharge. *Br Med J* **303**: 1023–6

Muijen M, Cooney M, Strathdee G, Bell R, Hudson A (1994) Community psychiatric nurse teams: intensive support versus generic care. *Br J Psychiatry* **165**: 211

Murphy D, Watters J (1986) Psychosis induced by fenfluramine. *Br Med J* **292**: 992

Nasrallah HA, Tolbert HA (1997) Neurobiology and neuroplasticity in schizophrenia — continuity across the life cycle. *Arch Gen Psychiatry* **54**: 913-4

Nelson HE, Thrasher S, Barnes TRE (1991) Practical ways of alleviating auditory hallucinations. *Br Med J* **302**: 327

Norman RMG, Malla AK (1993a) Stressful life events and schizophrenia. I: A review of the research. *Br J Psychiatry* **162**: 161–6

Norman RMG, Malla AK (1993b) Stressful life events and schizophrenia. II: Conceptual and methodological issues. *Br J Psychiatry* **162**: 166–74

Oldridge ML, Hughes ICT (1992) Psychological well-being in families with a member suffering from schizophrenia. An investigation into long-standing problems. *Br J Psychiatry* **161**: 249

Owens DGC (1990) Dystonia - a potential psychiatric pitfall. *Br J Psychiatry* **156**: 620

Parnas J, Schulsinger F, Schulsinger H, Mednick SA, Teasdale TW (1982) Behavioral precursors of schizophrenia spectrum. A prospective study. *Arch Gen Psychiatry* **39**: 658–64

Pickar D (1995) Prospects for pharmacotherapy of schizophrenia. *Lancet* **345**: 557–62

Ramsay M, Percy A (1996) *British Crime Survey 1994. Home Office Research Study 151.* Home Office, London

Reddy R, Mukherjee S, Schnur DB (1992) Comparison of negative symptoms in schizophrenic and poor outcome bipolar patients. *Psychol Med* **22**: 361–5

Regier D, Farmer M, Rae D (1990) Comorbidity of mental disorders with alcohol and other drug abuse. Results from the Epidemiological Catchment Area study. *J Am Med Ass* **264**: 2511–8

Rodriguez-Ferrera S, Vassilas CA (1998) Older people with schizophrenia: providing services for a neglected group. *Br Med J* **317**: 293–4

Rosenthal D, Wender PH, Kety SS, Welner J, Shulsinger F (1971) The adopted-away offspring of schizophrenics. *Am J Psychiatry* **128**: 307–11

Russell AJ, Munro JC, Jones PB, Hemsley DR, Murray RM (1997) Schizophrenia and the myth of intellectual decline. *Am J Psychiatry* **154**: 635–9

Scott DW, Wood RL (1987) The role of food substitutes in a token economy system. *Br J Psychiatry* **150**: 864

Scott J (1993) Homelessness and mental illness. *Br J Psychiatry* **162**: 314–24

Schneider K (1974) Primary and secondary symptoms in schizophrenia. In: Hirsch SR, Shepherd M, eds. *Themes and Variations in European Psychiatry.* J Wright, Bristol: 40–44

Sedvall G, Farde L (1995) Chemical brain anatomy in schizophrenia. *Lancet* **346**: 743–9

Seeman P, Lee T, Chau-Wong M, Wong K (1976) Antipsychotic drug doses and neuroleptic/ dopamine receptors. *Nature* **261**: 717–8

Shagass C, Roemer RA, Straumanis JJ (1982) Relationships between psychiatric diagnosis and some quantitative EEG variables. *Arch Gen Psychiatry* **39**: 1423–35

Sherrington R, Brynjolfsson J, Petursson H *et al* (1988) Localisation of a susceptibility locus for schizophrenia on chromosome 5. *Nature* **336**: 164–7

Sullivan G, Wells KB, Morgenstern H, Leake B (1995) Identifying modifiable risk factors for rehospitalization: a case-control study of seriously mentally ill persons in Mississippi. *Am J Psychiatry* **152**: 1749–56

Tarrier N, Yusupoff L, Kinney C *et al* (1988) Randomised controlled trial of intensive cognitive behaviour therapy for patients with chronic schizophrenia. *Br Med J* **317**: 303–7

Thomas H (1993) Psychiatric symptoms in cannabis users. *Br J Psychiatry* **163**: 141–9

Thomas P, Kearney G, Napier E, Ellis E, Leuder I, Johnson M (1996) Speech and language in first onset psychosis differences between people with schizophrenia, mania, and controls. *Br J Psychiatry* **168**: 337–43

Thornicroft G, Breakey WR (1991) The COSTAR programme. 1: Improving social networks of the long-term mentally ill. *Br J Psychiatry* **159**: 245–9

Vaughn CE, Leff JP (1976) The influence of family and social factors in the course of psychiatric illness. *Br J Psychiatry* **129**: 125–37

Verdoux H, Geddes JR, Takei N *et al* (1997) Obstetric Complications and Age at Onset in Schizophrenia: An International Collaborative Meta-Analysis of Individual Patient Data. *Am J Psychiatry* **154**: 1220–7

Waddington JL (1993) Schizophrenia: developmental neuroscience and pathobiology. *Lancet* **341**: 531–6

Walker EF, Grimes KE, Davis DM, Smith AJ (1993) Childhood precursors of schizophrenia: facial expression of emotion. *Am J Psychiatry* **150**: 1654-–0

White AJ, Barraclough B (1986) Radiology for psychiatric patients? *Br Med J* **292**: 800–1

White AJ, Barraclough B (1989) Benefits and problems of routine laboratory investigations in adult psychiatric admissions. *Br J Psychiatry* **155**: 65–72

WHO Heads of Centres collaborating in WHO co-ordinated studies on biological aspects of mental illness (1990) Prophylactic use of anticholinergics in patients on long-term neuroleptic treatment. A consensus statement. *Br J Psychiatry* **156**: 412

Wittenborn JR (1977) Stability of symptom ratings for schizophrenic men. *Arch Gen Psychiatry* **34**: 437–40

Wright P, Takei N, Rifkin L, Murray RM (1995) Maternal influenza, obstetric complications, and schizophrenia. *Am J Psychiatry* **152**: 1714–20

Further reading

APA Practice Guidelines for the Treatment of Patients with Schizophrenia. *Am J Psychiatry* April 1997

Index